TABLE OF CONTENTS

THE BRAIN HEALTHY COOKBOOK

Cleanses & Recipes For Neurological Health Fuel Your Brain, Heal Your Body, Unleashing the Healing Power of Food

Jessica M. Steven

INTRODUCTION

Welcome to the vibrant world of the Brain Healthy Cookbook, where the tantalizing aromas of wholesome ingredients and the promise of nourishing meals beckon you into a realm of culinary delight and cognitive wellness. As you step into this sacred space, allow me to guide you through the journey of nurturing not just your body, but also your most precious asset – your brain.

The Importance of Brain Health

The brain that marvel of evolution nestled snugly within our skulls, orchestrating the symphony of our thoughts, emotions, and actions. Our brain is not just a mere organ; it is the very essence of our being, the seat of our consciousness, and the gateway to our experiences. Its health and vitality are paramount,
for they dictate the quality of our lives and the depth of our interactions with the world around us.

Imagine, if you will, a garden teeming with life – lush greenery, vibrant blossoms, and buzzing insects. Just as a gardener tends to the soil, nourishing it with nutrients and care to yield a bountiful harvest, so too must we nurture our brains. For without proper nourishment, our cognitive garden may wither, leaving us susceptible to the weeds of cognitive decline and mental fog.

But fear not, for the path to vibrant brain health lies not in unattainable feats or esoteric rituals, but in the humble act of nourishing our bodies with the right foods and nutrients. Through mindful consumption and a dash of culinary creativity, we can cultivate a sanctuary of cognitive wellness within our very kitchens.

Using Nutrition to Support Cognitive Function
The alchemical art of transforming simple ingredients into nourishing elixirs for the body and soul. Just as a painter wields a brush to create a masterpiece on canvas, so too can we harness the power of food to paint a portrait of vibrant brain health.
Science has shown us that certain nutrients, omega-3 fatty acids, antioxidants, vitamins, and minerals – hold the key to unlocking our brain's full potential. From the humble blueberry, bursting with antioxidants to protect our neurons, to the mighty salmon, rich in omega-3s to fuel our cognitive engines, the bounty of nature offers us a cornucopia of treasures to support our mental acuity and emotional well-being.

By embracing a diet rich in whole, nutrient-dense foods, we can fortify our brains against the ravages of time and stress, empowering ourselves to navigate life's challenges with clarity and resilience. So let us raise our spatulas and apron strings in celebration of the wondrous journey that awaits us in the realm of brain-boosting cuisine.
How This Book Can Help
Now, you may be wondering, "How can this book assist me on my quest for brain health and culinary excellence?" Allow me to illuminate the path before you. Within these pages, you will find a treasure trove of delicious recipes, thoughtfully crafted to nourish your body and tantalize your taste buds.
From hearty breakfasts to soul-satisfying dinners, from energizing snacks to refreshing beverages, each recipe is meticulously designed to incorporate brain-boosting ingredients and culinary flair. But this book is more than just a collection of recipes; it is a roadmap to a lifestyle of cognitive wellness.
As you embark on this culinary adventure, you will not only feed your body but also nourish your mind and spirit. You will discover the joy of mindful eating, the pleasure of savoring each bite, and the satisfaction of knowing that you are fueling your brain for optimal performance.
So join me, as we journey together into the heart of the Brain Healthy Cookbook. Let us explore the boundless possibilities that await us, armed with spatulas, mixing bowls, and a hunger for knowledge. Together, we will unlock the secrets of culinary alchemy and pave the way to a brighter, sharper, and more vibrant future.

To illustrate the importance of brain health, let's consider the case of John, a middle-aged man who leads a sedentary lifestyle and consumes an unhealthy diet high in processed foods. John often struggles with forgetfulness and has difficulty centrating at work. He also experiences frequent mood swings and feels mentally exhausted most of the time.

Upon visiting his doctor, John learns that his poor brain health may be attributed to his lifestyle choices. His doctor explains that regular exercise stimulates blood flow to the brain, promoting the growth of new neurons and enhancing cognitive function. Additionally, consuming a nutrient-rich diet provides the necessary building blocks for optimal brain function.

Motivated by this information, John decides to make positive changes in his life. He starts incorporating regular exercise into his routine and adopts a brain-healthy diet rich in fruits, vegetables, whole grains, lean proteins, and healthy fats. Over time, John notices significant improvements in his memory, focus, and overall well-being.

To illustrate the connection between food and the brain, let's consider the case of Emma, a middle-aged woman who has been experiencing frequent migraines. Emma noticed that her migraines often occurred after consuming certain foods like processed meats and aged cheeses. Curious about this connection, she consulted a nutritionist.
The nutritionist explained to Emma that certain foods contain substances called tyramine and nitrates that can trigger migraines in susceptible individuals. Tyramine is found in aged cheeses, cured meats, and fermented foods, while nitrates are commonly found in processed meats like bacon and hot dogs. By avoiding these trigger foods and incorporating more fresh fruits, vegetables, whole grains, and lean proteins into her diet, Emma was able to significantly reduce the frequency and intensity of her migraines.

CHAPTER ONE
Understanding Brain Health

Anatomy and Function of the Brain
The marvel that is the human brain, a wondrous and intricate organ that serves as the command center of our bodies and the seat of our consciousness. As I delve into the depths of its anatomy and function, I am filled with awe and reverence for this remarkable masterpiece of nature.
Picture, if you will, a complex network of billions of neurons, each interconnected like the threads of a grand tapestry. These neurons form the building blocks of our thoughts, emotions, and actions, allowing us to perceive the world around us, form memories, and make decisions.

At the helm of this neuronal orchestra lies the brain's various regions, each tasked with specific functions essential to our daily lives. The frontal lobe, for instance, governs our higher cognitive functions, such as decision-making and problem-solving, while the temporal lobe plays a crucial role in memory formation and language processing. Meanwhile, the brainstem and cerebellum regulate our basic bodily functions, such as breathing, heart rate, and coordination.
But the brain is not merely a static organ; it is a dynamic and adaptable powerhouse that constantly evolves in response to our experiences and environment. Through a process known as neuroplasticity, our brains have the remarkable ability to reorganize and rewire themselves in response to learning, injury, and even aging.
This incredible adaptability underscores the importance of nurturing our brains throughout our lives, ensuring their continued vitality and resilience.

Factors Affecting Brain Health

As I reflect on the factors that influence the health and well-being of our brains, I am struck by the multifaceted nature of this intricate puzzle. Indeed, numerous factors both internal and external – play a role in shaping the health and vitality of our most precious organ.

Internal factors, such as genetics and age, undoubtedly influence our brain health, predisposing us to certain conditions and vulnerabilities. However, it is the external factors – our lifestyle choices, environment, and habits that often wield the greatest impact on our brain's longevity and resilience.

Consider, for example, the profound effects of stress on the brain. Chronic stress not only takes a toll on our mental and emotional well-being but also has tangible effects on the structure and function of the brain itself. Prolonged exposure to stress hormones, such as cortisol, can lead to shrinkage of the hippocampus, the brain's memory center – and impair our ability to learn and remember.

Similarly, inadequate sleep, poor nutrition, and sedentary lifestyles can all contribute to cognitive decline and increase our risk of neurodegenerative diseases, such as Alzheimer's and Parkinson's. However, by making conscious choices to prioritize our brain health through regular exercise, healthy eating, and stress management techniques we can mitigate these risks and optimize our brain's potential for resilience and vitality.

The Connection Between Nutrition and Cognitive Function

The age-old adage "you are what you eat" rings true, especially when it comes to our brain health. As I explore the intricate web of connections between nutrition and cognitive function, I am struck by the profound impact that our dietary choices can have on the health and vitality of our brains. Consider, for instance, the role of omega-3 fatty acids those essential nutrients found abundantly in fatty fish, nuts, and seeds. These fatty acids are not only integral to the structure of our brain cell membranes but also play a crucial role in neurotransmission the communication between brain cells. By incorporating omega-3-rich foods into our diets, we can support healthy brain function and protect against cognitive decline.

Similarly, antioxidants those powerful compounds found in colorful fruits and vegetables – play a vital role in protecting our brains from oxidative stress and inflammation. These antioxidants, such as vitamins C and E, help neutralize harmful free radicals that can damage brain cells and contribute to age-related cognitive decline.

Furthermore, certain vitamins and minerals – such as vitamin B12, folate, and iron are essential for the production of neurotransmitters, the chemical messengers that relay signals between brain cells. By ensuring adequate intake of these nutrients through a varied and balanced diet, we can support optimal brain function and mental clarity.

In conclusion, the connection between nutrition and cognitive function is undeniable. By nourishing our bodies with a diet rich in whole, nutrient-dense foods, we can fuel our brains for optimal performance and protect against the ravages of time and stress. So let us savor each bite, mindful of the profound impact it has on our most precious organ, our brain.

CHAPTER TWO
Key Nutrients for Brain Health

Highlighting Essential Nutrients for Brain Health

As I delve into the realm of essential nutrients that support our brain's magnificent function, I am filled with a sense of wonder at the intricate interplay between food and cognitive vitality. Let us embark on a journey of discovery, exploring the roles of omega-3 fatty acids, antioxidants, vitamins, and minerals in nurturing our brain health, and uncovering the bountiful sources of these nutrients that nature has bestowed upon us.

Omega-3 Fatty Acids: Nourishing the Brain's Building Blocks

Omega-3 fatty acids, those mighty warriors of brain health, revered for their ability to fortify our neural architecture and enhance cognitive function. As I contemplate their importance, I am reminded of the vast oceans from which these essential fatty acids derive their power, as well as the humble seeds and nuts that harbor their nourishing bounty.

Omega-3 fatty acids, particularly EPA (eicosapentaenoic acid) and DHA (docosahexaenoic acid), are integral components of our brain cell membranes, providing structural support and fluidity essential for optimal neural communication. Moreover, these fatty acids possess anti-inflammatory properties, safeguarding our brains against the ravages of oxidative stress and inflammation.

Sources of omega-3 fatty acids abound in nature, from fatty fish such as salmon, mackerel, and sardines, to plant-based sources like flaxseeds, chia seeds, and walnuts. By incorporating these omega-3-rich foods into our diets, we can nourish our brains and protect against cognitive decline.

Antioxidants Nature's Guardians of Brain Health

As I marvel at the vibrant hues of nature's bounty from ruby-red berries to emerald-green leafy greens I am reminded of the potent antioxidants that lie within, safeguarding our brains against oxidative damage and preserving cognitive function.

Antioxidants, such as vitamin C, vitamin E, and various phytonutrients, neutralize harmful free radicals that can wreak havoc on our brain cells, protecting against age-related cognitive decline and neurodegenerative diseases. Moreover, these antioxidants promote healthy blood flow to the brain, enhancing nutrient delivery and waste removal.

Sources of antioxidants are plentiful and diverse, ranging from colorful fruits and vegetables like berries, citrus fruits, spinach, and kale, to antioxidant-rich beverages such as green tea and dark chocolate. By embracing a rainbow of plant-based foods, we can flood our bodies with these protective compounds and nurture our brains for optimal health.

Vitamins and Minerals: Essential Nutrients for Cognitive Vitality

The vitamins and minerals that serve as the building blocks of our cognitive vitality they are the unsung heroes of brain health, tirelessly supporting our mental acuity and emotional well-being. From the vitamin-rich fruits and vegetables that grace our tables to the mineral rich grains and legumes that nourish our bodies, these essential nutrients are the lifeblood of our brain's resilience.

Vitamins such as B vitamins (including B12, folate, and B6) play crucial roles in neurotransmitter synthesis, ensuring efficient communication between brain cells and supporting mood regulation and cognitive function. Meanwhile, minerals such as iron, zinc, and magnesium are vital for oxygen transport, enzyme activity, and synaptic plasticity, facilitating learning and memory.

Sources of vitamins and minerals are abundant in a varied and balanced diet, encompassing a wide array of foods such as lean meats, poultry, fish, dairy products, whole grains, legumes, nuts, seeds, fruits, and vegetables. By prioritizing nutrient-dense foods in our daily meals, we can nourish our brains with the vitamins and minerals essential for optimal cognitive health.

Tips for Incorporating Brain-Boosting Nutrients Into Daily Meals

As we navigate the culinary landscape in search of brain-boosting nutrients, let us not forget the simple pleasures of wholesome cooking and mindful eating.

Here are some tips to help you incorporate these essential nutrients into your daily meals:

1. Start your day with a brain-boosting breakfast, such as a hearty bowl of oatmeal topped with walnuts and berries, or a salmon and avocado breakfast sandwich on whole-grain bread.

2. Incorporate omega-3-rich foods into your diet by enjoying fatty fish at least twice a week, adding ground flaxseeds or chia seeds to smoothies and oatmeal, or snacking on a handful of walnuts.

3. Load up on antioxidant-rich fruits and vegetables by filling half your plate with colorful produce at each meal. Enjoy antioxidant-packed snacks like sliced bell peppers with hummus or a mixed berry smoothie.

4. Boost your intake of vitamins and minerals by incorporating a variety of nutrient-dense foods into your meals, such as leafy greens, citrus fruits, nuts, seeds, whole grains, and lean proteins.

5. Experiment with herbs and spices like turmeric, cinnamon, and ginger, which not only add flavor to your dishes but also boast antioxidant and anti-inflammatory properties.

By embracing these simple strategies and savoring the abundance of nature's bounty, we can nourish our brains with the essential nutrients they need to thrive. So let us embark on this culinary adventure with joy and curiosity, knowing that each meal we share nourishes not only our bodies but also our minds.

CHAPTER THREE
Building a Brain Healthy Kitchen

Practical Advice for Stocking a Brain-Boosting Kitchen
As I open the doors to my kitchen, I am filled with anticipation and excitement, knowing that within these walls lie the building blocks of my cognitive vitality. Join me as I share practical advice for stocking your pantry and fridge with brain-boosting ingredients, offering tips for meal planning and preparation, and suggesting kitchen tools and gadgets to aid in your culinary endeavors.

Stocking Your Pantry and Fridge
The first step in creating a brain-boosting kitchen is to ensure that your pantry and fridge are stocked with nutrient-dense ingredients that support cognitive health. Here are some essential items to include:

1. Whole Grains Option for whole grains such as brown rice, quinoa, oats, and whole wheat pasta, which are rich in fiber and essential nutrients like B vitamins and magnesium.

2. Healthy Fats Incorporate sources of healthy fats such as olive oil, avocado oil, nuts, seeds, and fatty fish like salmon and mackerel, which provide omega-3 fatty acids essential for brain health.

3. Colorful Fruits and Vegetables Fill your fridge with a rainbow of fruits and vegetables, including berries, leafy greens, cruciferous vegetables, and citrus fruits, which are packed with antioxidants, vitamins, and minerals.

4. Lean Proteins Include lean proteins like chicken, turkey, tofu, and legumes, which provide amino acids necessary for neurotransmitter synthesis and muscle repair.

5. Herbs and Spices Keep a variety of herbs and spices on hand, such as turmeric, ginger, cinnamon, and rosemary, which not only add flavor to your dishes but also boast antioxidant and anti-inflammatory properties.

By stocking your pantry and fridge with these brain-boosting ingredients, you can ensure that you have the building blocks necessary to create nutritious and delicious meals that support cognitive function.

Meal Planning and Preparation Tips

Meal planning and preparation are essential components of maintaining a brain-healthy diet amidst the hustle and bustle of daily life. Here are some tips to make cooking nutritious meals easier and more convenient.

1. Plan Ahead Set aside some time each week to plan your meals and create a shopping list based on the ingredients you already have on hand and what you need to replenish.

2. Batch Cooking Consider batch cooking staple items like grains, beans, and proteins in large quantities, then portioning them out for easy meal assembly throughout the week.

3. Prep Ingredients in Advance Wash, chop, and portion out fruits, vegetables, and other ingredients in advance, so they're ready to use when you need them.

4. Use Time-Saving Cooking Methods Option for time-saving cooking methods like one-pot meals, sheet pan dinners, and slow cooker recipes, which require minimal hands-on time and yield delicious results.

5. Freeze Extras If you make larger batches of meals or components, consider freezing extras for future meals, ensuring that you always have nutritious options on hand, even on busy days.

By incorporating these meal planning and preparation tips into your routine, you can streamline the cooking process and make it easier to stick to a brain-healthy diet.

Kitchen tools and gadgets that can make preparing brain-healthy Cooking

In addition to stocking your kitchen with brain-boosting ingredients and mastering meal planning and preparation, having the right tools and gadgets can also aid in your culinary endeavors. Here are some kitchen tools and gadgets that can make preparing brain-healthy recipes even easier.

1. High-Speed Blender A high-speed blender is a versatile tool that can be used to whip up smoothies, soups, sauces, and nut butters, making it easy to incorporate fruits, vegetables, and nuts into your diet.

2. Food Processor A food processor is perfect for chopping, slicing, and shredding fruits, vegetables, nuts, and seeds, saving you time and effort in the kitchen.

3. Steamer Basket A steamer basket is a convenient way to cook vegetables while preserving their nutrients, ensuring that they retain their vibrant colors and flavors.

4. Instant Pot An Instant Pot is a multipurpose electric pressure cooker that can be used to cook grains, beans, soups, stews, and more in a fraction of the time compared to traditional cooking methods.

5. Mandoline Slicer A mandoline slicer allows you to quickly and evenly slice fruits and vegetables with precision, making it easier to incorporate them into your meals.

By investing in these kitchen tools and gadgets, you can streamline the cooking process and make it even easier to prepare nutritious and delicious meals that support cognitive health.

In conclusion, stocking your pantry and fridge with brain-boosting ingredients, mastering meal planning and preparation, and investing in the right kitchen tools and gadgets are essential steps in creating a brain-healthy kitchen. By incorporating these practical tips into your culinary routine, you can nourish your brain and support optimal cognitive function for years to come.

Breakfasts for Brain Power
Energizing Smoothie Bowls
Nutrient-Packed Oatmeal
Variations
Protein-Packed Breakfast
Burritos
Brain-Boosting Breakfast
Bakes

Berry Blast Smoothie Bowl

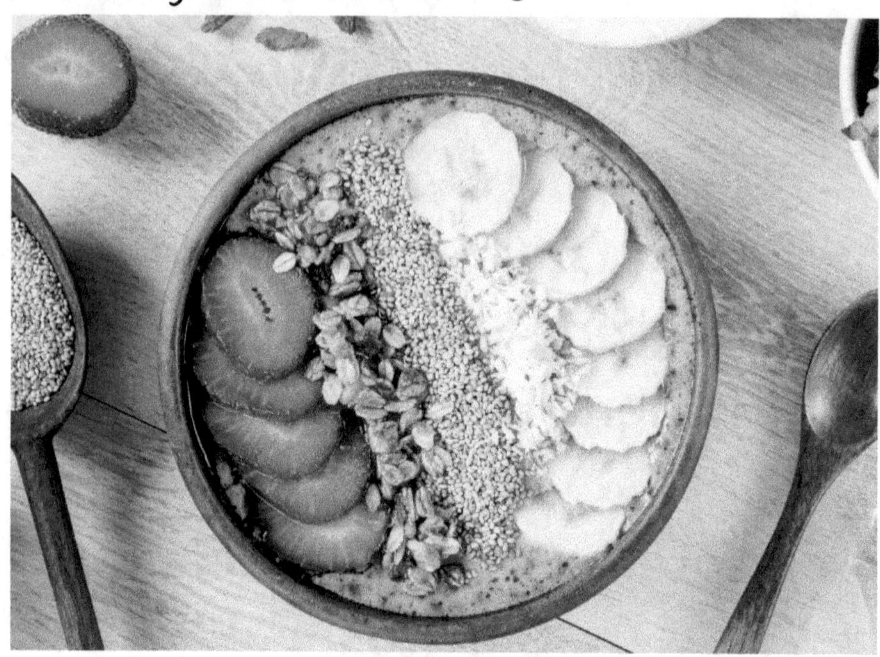

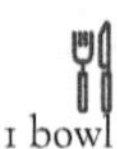

1 bowl   **5 minutes**

INGREDIENTS

1 frozen banana

1/2 cup mixed berries (such as strawberries, blueberries, and raspberries)

1 cup fresh spinach leaves

1/2 cup almond milk

1 tablespoon chia seeds

Toppings of your choice (e.g., sliced fruit, granola, nuts, seeds)

NUTRITIONAL VALUE

100 ml milk

50 g butter

3 eggs

1 tbs cocoa

2 tsp baking soda

a pinch of salt

3 eggs

DIRECTIONS

1. 1. In a blender, combine frozen banana, mixed berries, spinach, almond milk, and chia seeds.
2. 2. Blend until smooth and creamy.
3. 3. Pour into a bowl and add your favorite toppings.
4. 4. Serve immediately and enjoy!

DESCRIPTION

This vibrant and refreshing smoothie bowl is bursting with the goodness of mixed berries, bananas, and spinach, providing a nourishing and energizing start to your day.

Tropical Paradise Smoothie Bowl

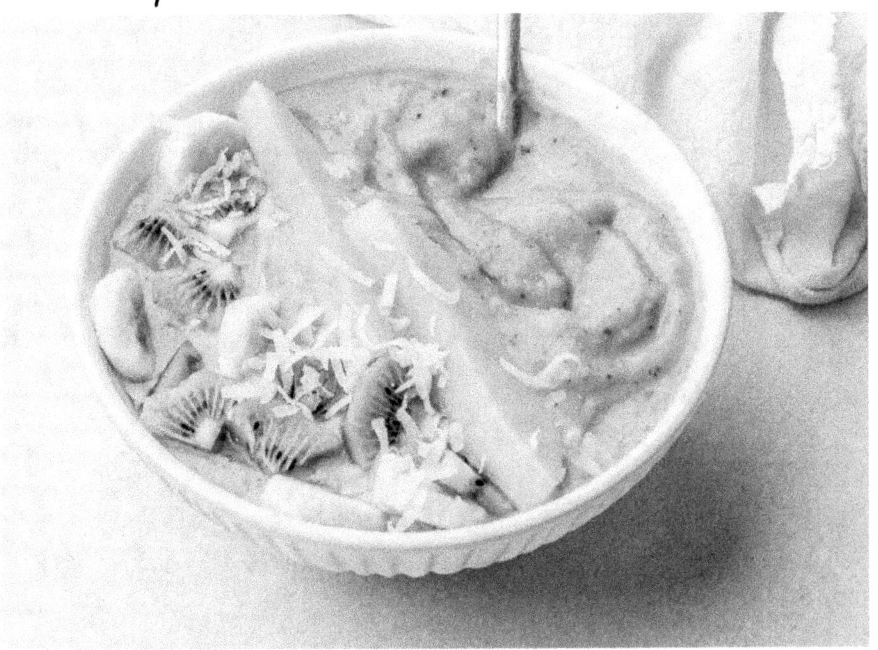

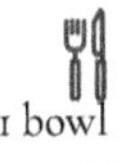 

1 bowl   5 minutes

INGREDIENTS

1/2 ripe mango, diced

1/2 cup frozen pineapple chunks

1/2 frozen banana

1/2 cup coconut water

1/4 cup plain Greek yogurt

1 tablespoon shredded coconut

Toppings of your choice (e.g., sliced mango, toasted coconut flakes, chia seeds)

NUTRITIONAL VALUE

Approximately 300 calories, 8g protein, 6g fat, 50g carbohydrates, 10g fiber.

DIRECTIONS

1. 1. In a blender, combine diced mango, frozen pineapple, frozen banana, coconut water, and Greek yogurt.

2. 2. Blend until smooth and creamy.

3. 3. Pour into a bowl and sprinkle with shredded coconut.

4. 4. Add your favorite toppings and serve immediately.

DESCRIPTION

Transport yourself to a tropical paradise with this delicious smoothie bowl featuring mango, pineapple, coconut, and banana, providing a burst of sunshine in every spoonful.

Apple Cinnamon Oatmeal

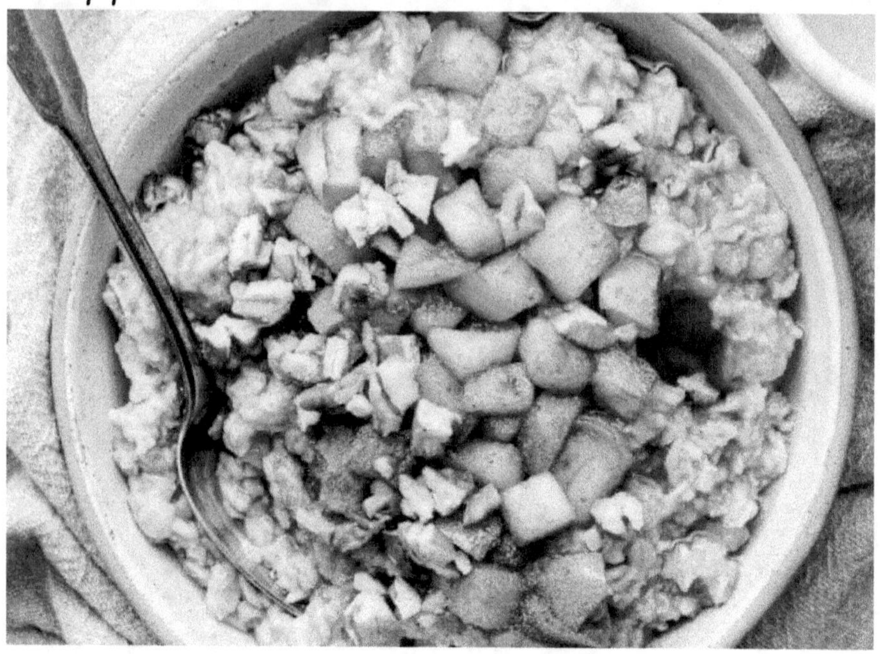

🍴 1 servings   🕐 10 minutes

INGREDIENTS

1/2 cup rolled oats
1 cup unsweetened almond milk
1 small apple, diced
1/2 teaspoon ground cinnamon
1 tablespoon maple syrup or
honey (optional)
Toppings of your choice (e.g.,
chopped nuts, dried fruit,
cinnamon)

NUTRITIONAL VALUE

100 ml milk
50 g butter
3 eggs
1 tbs cocoa
2 tsp baking soda
a pinch of salt
3 eggs

DIRECTIONS

1.1. In a saucepan, combine rolled oats, almond milk, diced apple, cinnamon, and maple syrup or honey (if using).

2.2. Bring to a simmer over medium heat, stirring occasionally.

3.3. Cook for 5-7 minutes, or until oats are tender and mixture has thickened.

4.4. Remove from heat and let cool slightly.

5.5. Transfer oatmeal to a bowl and add your favorite toppings.

6.6. Serve warm and enjoy!

DESCRIPTION

Warm and comforting, this apple cinnamon oatmeal is a classic breakfast favorite, infused with cozy spices and sweetened with fresh apples for a nutritious and satisfying meal.

Banana Nut Oatmeal

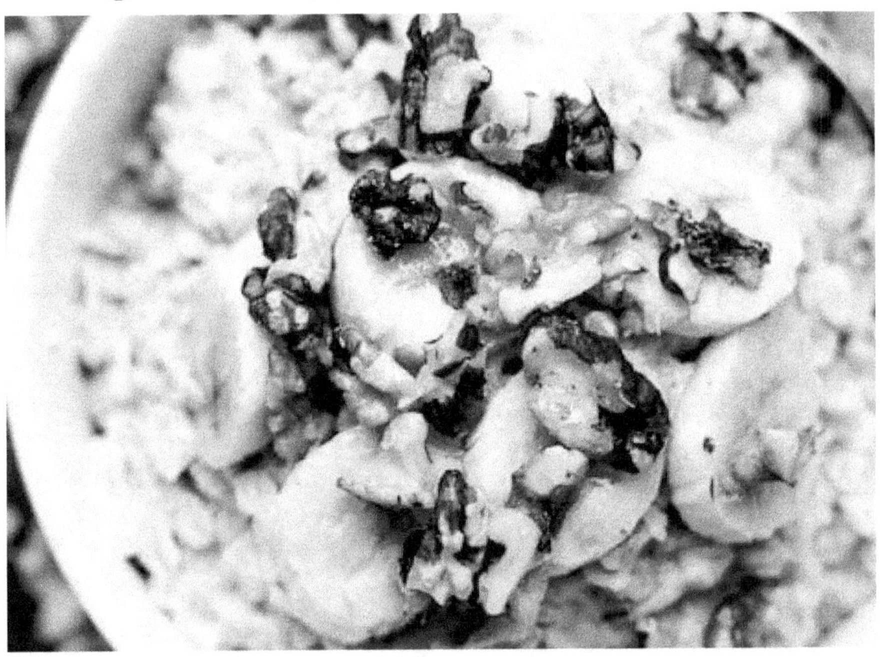

1 servings   10 minutes

INGREDIENTS

1/2 cup rolled oats

1 cup unsweetened almond milk

1 ripe banana, mashed

2 tablespoons chopped nuts (such as almonds or walnuts)

1 tablespoon maple syrup or honey (optional)

Toppings of your choice (e.g., sliced banana, additional nuts, cinnamon)

NUTRITIONAL VALUE

300 calories,

8g protein,

10g fat,

45g carbohydrates,

7g fiber

DIRECTIONS

1. 1. In a saucepan, combine rolled oats, almond milk, mashed banana, chopped nuts, and maple syrup or honey (if using).

2. 2. Bring to a simmer over medium heat, stirring occasionally.

3. 3. Cook for 5-7 minutes, or until oats are tender and mixture has thickened.

4. 4. Remove from heat and let cool slightly.

5. 5. Transfer oatmeal to a bowl and add your favorite toppings.

6. 6. Serve warm and enjoy!

DESCRIPTION

Creamy and satisfying, this banana nut oatmeal is filled with the natural sweetness of ripe bananas and the crunch of chopped nuts, making it a hearty and nutritious breakfast option.

Veggie and Egg Breakfast Burrito

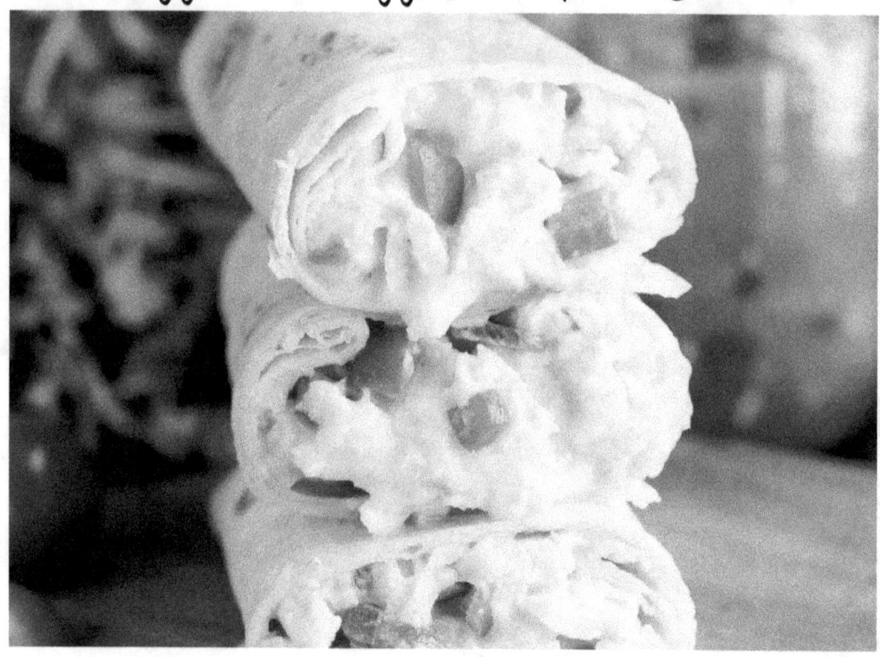

1 burrito

15 minutes

INGREDIENTS

1 large whole wheat or spinach
tortilla

2 large eggs, scrambled

1/4 cup chopped bell peppers

1/4 cup chopped onions

1/4 cup sliced mushrooms

1/4 ripe avocado, sliced

Salsa or hot sauce for serving

NUTRITIONAL VALUE

400 calories,

20g protein,

15g fat,

45g carbohydrates,

8g fiber.

DIRECTIONS

1.1. In a skillet, sauté chopped bell peppers, onions, and mushrooms until tender.

2.2. Add scrambled eggs to the skillet and cook until set.

3.3. Warm tortilla in the microwave or on a skillet.

4.4. Spoon scrambled eggs and sautéed vegetables onto the center of the tortilla.

5.5. Top with sliced avocado and salsa or hot sauce, if desired.

6.6. Fold in the sides of the tortilla and roll up tightly.

7.7. Serve immediately and enjoy!

DESCRIPTION

Kickstart your day with this hearty and flavorful breakfast burrito filled with scrambled eggs, sautéed vegetables, and creamy avocado for a satisfying morning meal.

Blueberry Banana Breakfast Bake

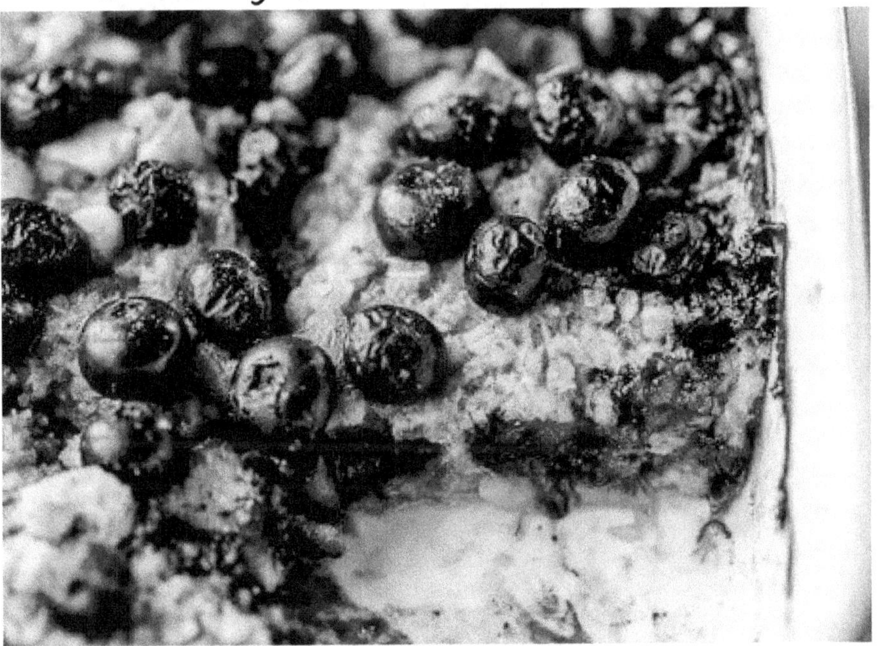

🍴 1 slice   🕐 40 minutes

INGREDIENTS

2 ripe bananas, mashed

1/2 cup unsweetened applesauce

1/4 cup maple syrup or honey

2 cups rolled oats

1 teaspoon baking powder

1/2 teaspoon cinnamon

1/2 cup fresh or frozen blueberries

Optional toppings: sliced bananas,
chopped nuts, maple syrup

NUTRITIONAL VALUE

200 calories,

5g protein,

3g fat,

40g carbohydrates,

6g fiber.

DIRECTIONS

1. 1. Preheat the oven to 350°F (175°C). Grease a baking dish with cooking spray or coconut oil.
2. 2. In a large bowl, combine mashed bananas, applesauce, and maple syrup or honey.
3. 3. Add rolled oats, baking powder, and cinnamon, and mix until well combined.
4. 4. Gently fold in blueberries.
5. 5. Pour the mixture into the prepared baking dish and spread evenly.
6. 6. Bake for 30-35 minutes, or until golden brown and set.
7. 7. Allow to cool slightly before slicing.
8. 8. Serve warm, topped with sliced bananas, chopped nuts, and a drizzle of maple syrup, if desired.

DESCRIPTION

This delicious and nutritious breakfast bake is filled with the goodness of ripe bananas and juicy blueberries, making it a perfect make-ahead option for busy mornings.

Spinach and Feta Breakfast Quiche

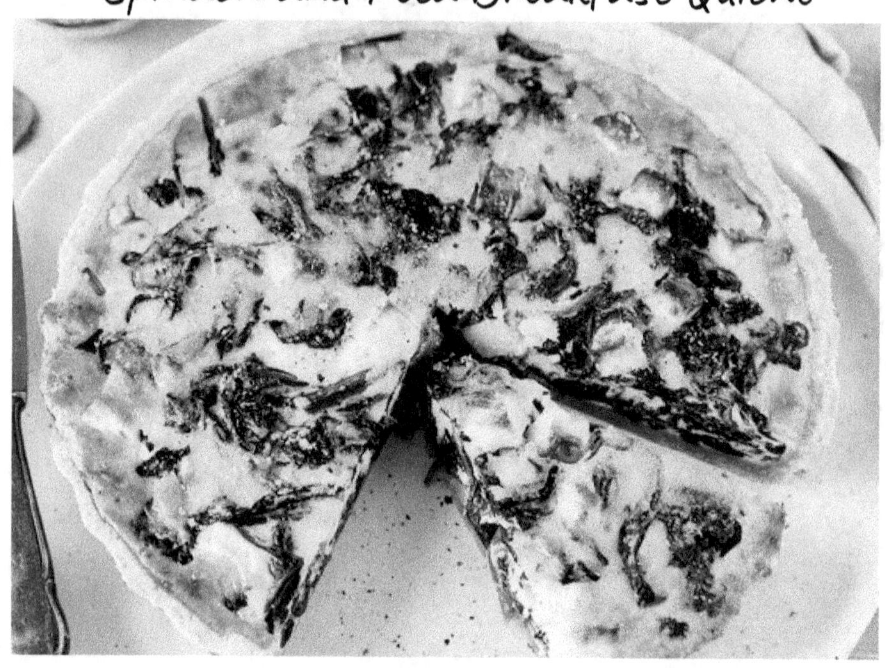

1 slice · **45 minutes**

INGREDIENTS

1 prepared pie crust (store-bought or homemade)

6 large eggs

1 cup unsweetened almond milk

2 cups fresh spinach, chopped

1/2 cup crumbled feta cheese

1/4 cup chopped sun-dried tomatoes

1/4 cup chopped green onions

Salt and pepper to taste

NUTRITIONAL VALUE

250 calories,

12g protein,

15g fat,

20g carbohydrates,

3g fiber.

DIRECTIONS

1. 1. Preheat the oven to 375°F (190°C). Place the pie crust in a pie dish and crimp the edges.
2. 2. In a large bowl, whisk together eggs and almond milk.
3. 3. Stir in chopped spinach, crumbled feta cheese, sun-dried tomatoes, green onions, salt, and pepper.
4. 4. Pour the egg mixture into the prepared pie crust.
5. 5. Bake for 30-35 minutes, or until the quiche is set and the crust is golden brown.
6. 6. Allow to cool slightly before slicing and serving.

DESCRIPTION

This savory breakfast quiche is loaded with nutrient-rich spinach, creamy feta cheese, and flavorful herbs, making it a perfect option for brunch gatherings or meal prep.

Peanut Butter Banana Breakfast Cookies

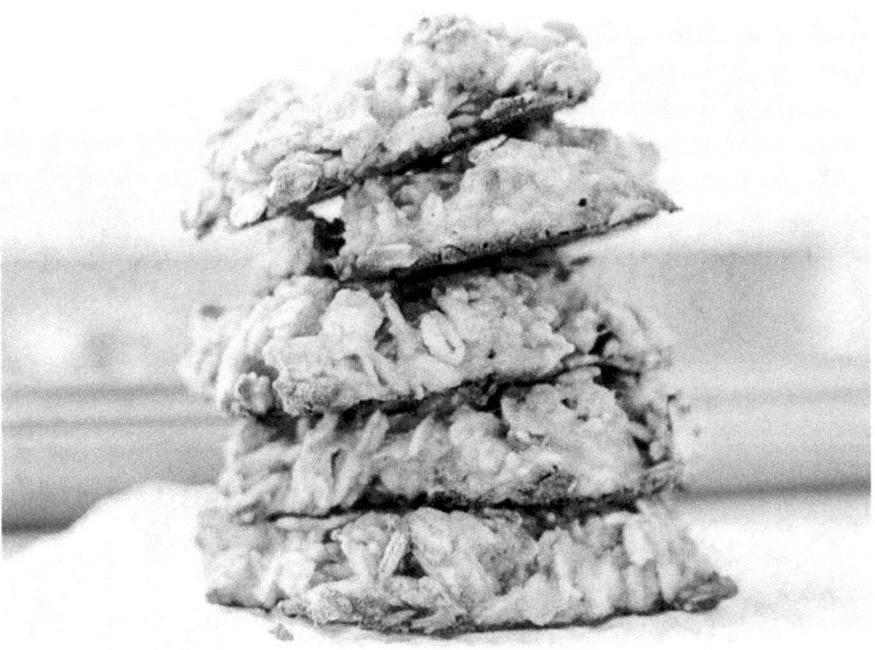

1 cookie   25 minutes

INGREDIENTS

2 ripe bananas, mashed

1/2 cup peanut butter

1/4 cup honey or maple syrup

2 cups rolled oats

1 teaspoon vanilla extract

1/2 teaspoon cinnamon

1/4 cup dark chocolate chips (optional)

NUTRITIONAL VALUE

150 calories,

4g protein,

8g fat,

18g carbohydrates,

2g fiber.

DIRECTIONS

1. 1. Preheat the oven to 350°F (175°C). Line a baking sheet with parchment paper.
2. 2. In a large bowl, combine mashed bananas, peanut butter, honey or maple syrup, rolled oats, vanilla extract, and cinnamon.
3. 3. Stir until well combined. If using, fold in dark chocolate chips.
4. 4. Drop spoonfuls of dough onto the prepared baking sheet, and flatten slightly with the back of a spoon.
5. 5. Bake for 12–15 minutes, or until golden brown.
6. 6. Allow to cool on the baking sheet for 5 minutes before transferring to a wire rack to cool completely.

DESCRIPTION

These delicious breakfast cookies are packed with wholesome ingredients like oats, bananas, and peanut butter, making them a nutritious and portable option for busy mornings.

Mediterranean Egg Muffins

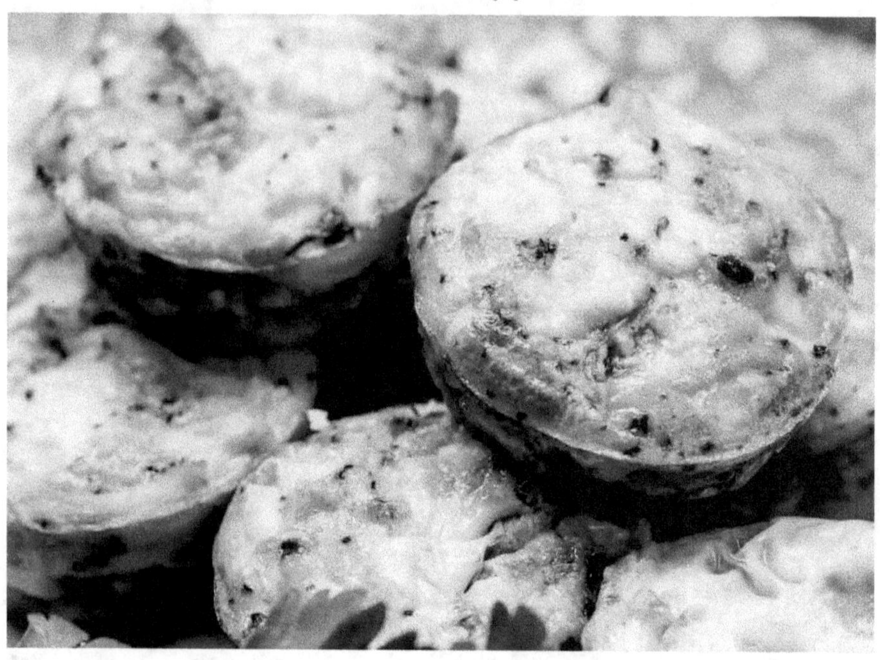

2 egg muffins

25 minutes

INGREDIENTS

6 large eggs

1/4 cup unsweetened almond milk

1/2 cup chopped spinach

1/4 cup diced tomatoes

1/4 cup sliced black olives

1/4 cup crumbled feta cheese

Salt and pepper to taste

Fresh parsley for garnish (optional

DIRECTIONS

200 calories,

12g protein,

12g fat,

5g carbohydrates,

1g fiber.

DIRECTIONS

1.1. Preheat the oven to 350°F (175°C). Grease a muffin tin with cooking spray or line with muffin liners.

2.2. In a large bowl, whisk together eggs and almond milk.

3.3. Stir in chopped spinach, diced tomatoes, sliced black olives, crumbled feta cheese, salt, and pepper.

4.4. Pour the egg mixture evenly into the prepared muffin tin.

5.5. Bake for 15-18 minutes, or until eggs are set and lightly golden.

6.6. Allow to cool slightly before serving.

7.7. Garnish with fresh parsley, if desired.

DIRECTIONS

These Mediterranean-inspired egg muffins are filled with savory ingredients like tomatoes, spinach, olives, and feta cheese, making them a perfect grab-and-go breakfast option.

Sweet Potato and Kale Breakfast Hash

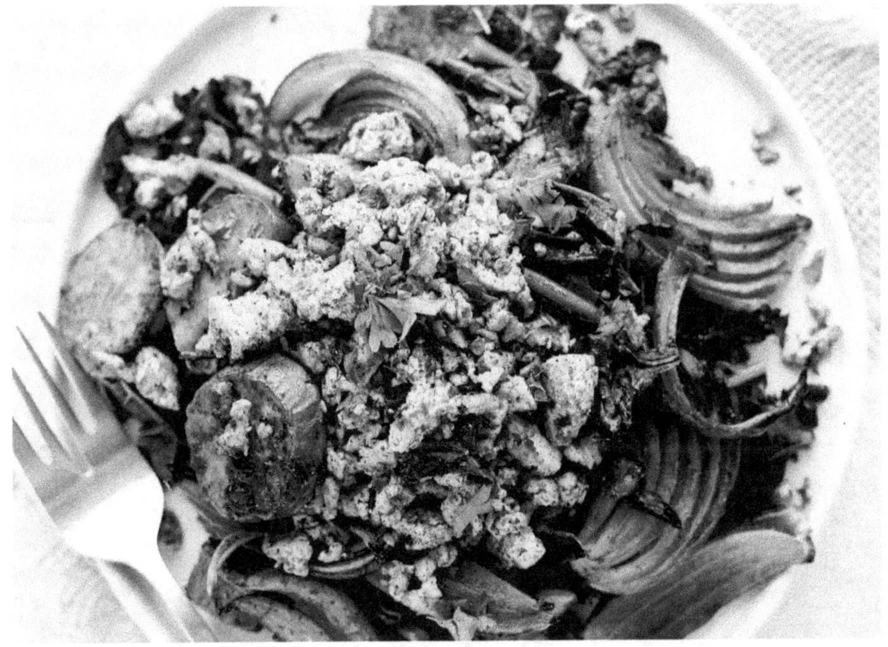

1 servings   **30 minutes**

INGREDIENTS

1 large sweet potato, diced

1 tablespoon olive oil

1/2 small onion, diced

1 cup chopped kale

2 large eggs

Salt and pepper to taste

Fresh parsley for garnish (optional)

DIRECTIONS

300 calories,

12g protein,

12g fat,

35g carbohydrates,

7g fiber.

DIRECTIONS

1. 1. Heat olive oil in a skillet over medium heat.
2. 2. Add diced sweet potato to the skillet and cook until tender and lightly browned, about 10-12 minutes.
3. 3. Add diced onion and chopped kale to the skillet and cook until kale is wilted and onions are translucent, about 5 minutes.
4. 4. Make two wells in the hash and crack an egg into each well.
5. 5. Cover and cook until eggs are set to your liking, about 5 minutes for runny yolks or longer for firmer yolks.
6. 6. Season with salt and pepper to taste.
7. 7. Garnish with fresh parsley, if desired, before serving.

DIRECTIONS

This hearty and satisfying breakfast hash features sweet potatoes, kale, onions, and eggs, providing a delicious and nutritious way to start your day.

Energizing Lunches
Colorful Grain Salads
Wholesome Wrap and Sandwich Creations
Satisfying Soup and Stew Recipes
Vibrant Buddha Bowls

Mediterranean Quinoa Salad

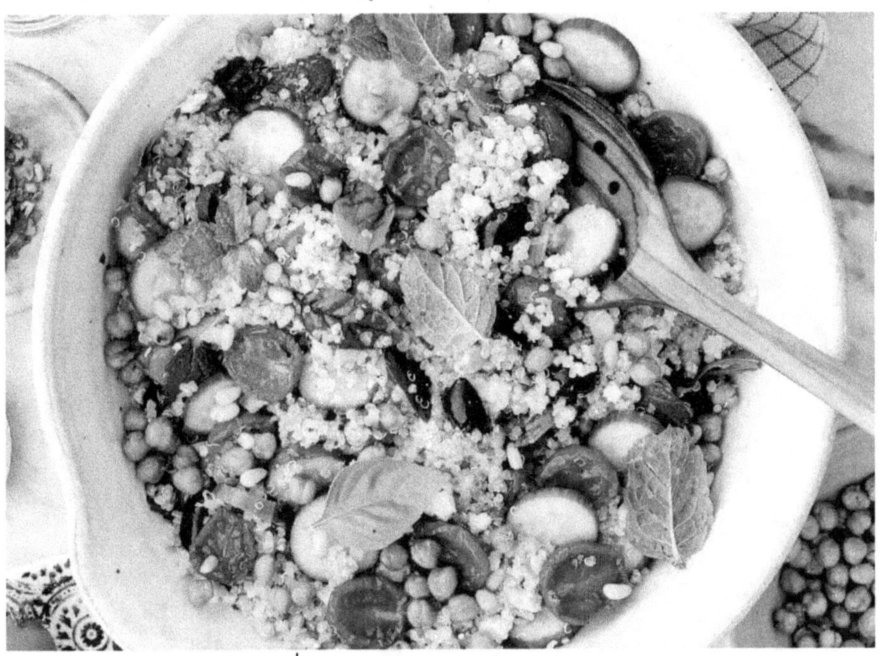

🍴 2 servings 🕐 20 minutes

INGREDIENTS

1 cup cooked quinoa
1 cup cherry tomatoes, halved
1/2 English cucumber, diced
1/4 cup sliced Kalamata olives
1/4 cup crumbled feta cheese
2 tablespoons chopped fresh parsley
2 tablespoons extra virgin olive oil
1 tablespoon freshly squeezed lemon juice
1 teaspoon dried oregano
Salt and pepper to taste

NUTRITIONAL VALUE

300 calories,
8g protein,
15g fat,
35g carbohydrates,
6g fiber.

DIRECTIONS

1. 1. In a large bowl, combine cooked quinoa, cherry tomatoes, cucumber, olives, feta cheese, and chopped parsley.
2. 2. In a small bowl, whisk together olive oil, lemon juice, dried oregano, salt, and pepper to make the dressing.
3. 3. Pour the dressing over the salad and toss gently to combine.
4. 4. Divide the salad into bowls and serve immediately, or refrigerate until ready to eat.

DESCRIPTION

This colorful and flavorful grain salad is inspired by the vibrant flavors of the Mediterranean, featuring quinoa, cherry tomatoes, cucumbers, olives, feta cheese, and a zesty lemon-herb dressing.

Veggie Hummus Wrap

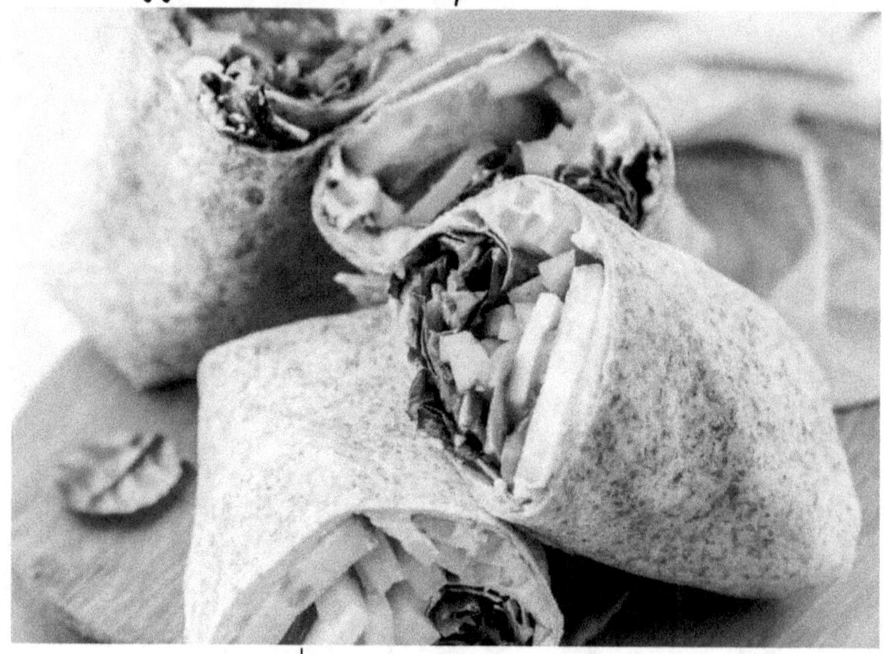

1 wrap

15 minutes

INGREDIENTS

1 large whole wheat or spinach
tortilla

2 tablespoons hummus

1/4 cup shredded carrots

1/4 cup sliced cucumbers

1/4 cup baby spinach leaves

1/4 cup diced red bell pepper

2 tablespoons crumbled feta
cheese

NUTRITIONAL VALUE

250 calories,

8g protein,

10g fat,

30g carbohydrates,

5g fiber.

DIRECTIONS

1. 1. Spread hummus evenly over the tortilla.
2. 2. Layer shredded carrots, sliced cucumbers, baby spinach leaves, diced red bell pepper, and crumbled feta cheese on top of the hummus.
3. 3. Roll up the tortilla tightly, folding in the sides as you go.
4. 4. Slice the wrap in half diagonally and serve immediately, or wrap tightly in foil for later.

DESCRIPTION

This wholesome and satisfying
wrap is filled with colorful
vegetables, creamy hummus, and
tangy feta cheese, making it a
perfect grab-and-go lunch option.

Lentil and Vegetable Soup

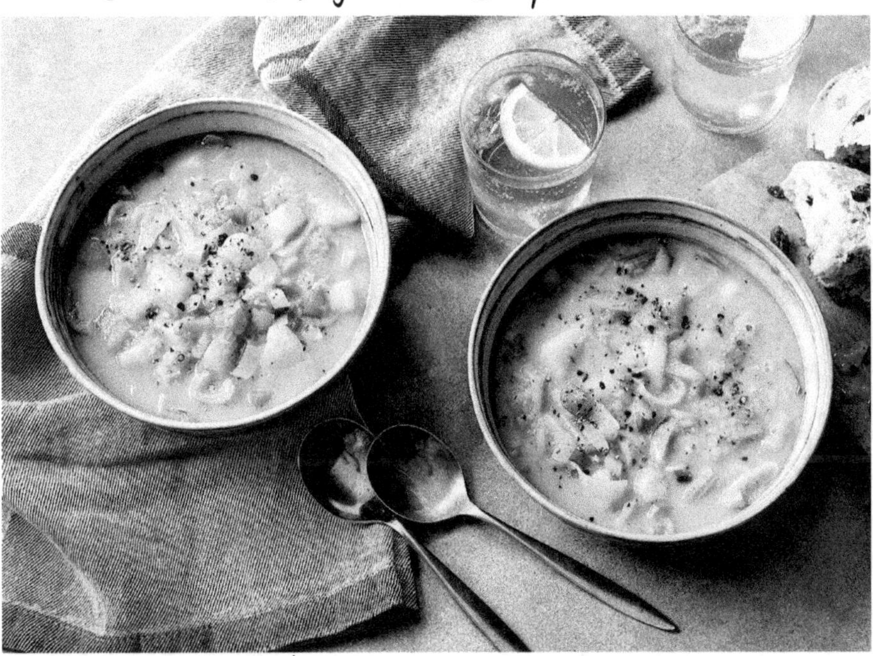

 2 servings

 30 minutes

INGREDIENTS

1 tablespoon olive oil

1/2 onion, diced

2 cloves garlic, minced

2 carrots, diced

2 celery stalks, diced

1/2 cup dried green or brown lentils, rinsed

4 cups vegetable broth

1 teaspoon ground cumin

1/2 teaspoon smoked paprika

Salt and pepper to taste

Fresh parsley for garnish (optional)

NUTRITIONAL VALUE

200 calories,

10g protein,

5g fat,

30g carbohydrates,

8g fiber.

DIRECTIONS

1.1. Heat olive oil in a large pot over medium heat.

2.2. Add diced onion and minced garlic, and cook until softened, about 5 minutes.

3.3. Add diced carrots and celery, and cook for another 5 minutes.

4.4. Stir in rinsed lentils, vegetable broth, ground cumin, smoked paprika, salt, and pepper.

5.5. Bring the soup to a boil, then reduce heat to low and simmer for 20-25 minutes, or until lentils are tender.

6.6. Taste and adjust seasoning as needed.

7.7. Ladle the soup into bowls, garnish with fresh parsley if desired, and serve hot.

DESCRIPTION

This hearty and nutritious soup is packed with protein-rich lentils, colorful vegetables, and aromatic spices, making it a satisfying meal-in-a-bowl for lunchtime.

Rainbow Veggie Buddha Bowl

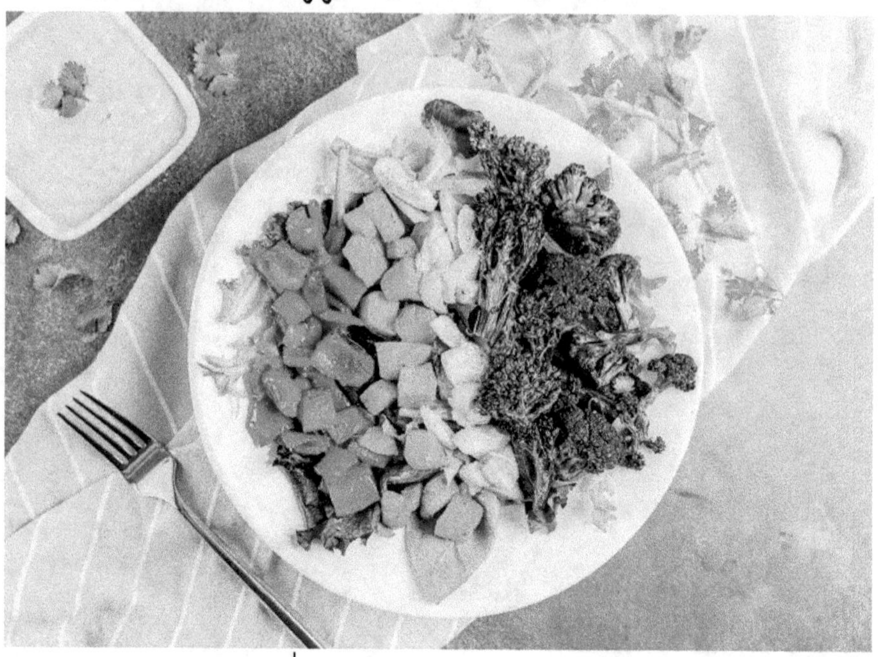

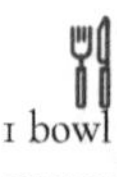 

1 bowl   30 minutes

INGREDIENTS

1 cup cooked quinoa or brown rice

1/2 cup cooked chickpeas

1/2 cup shredded purple cabbage

1/2 cup sliced bell peppers (assorted colors)

1/2 cup shredded carrots

1/2 cup cherry tomatoes, halved

1/2 avocado, sliced

2 tablespoons tahini

1 tablespoon freshly squeezed lemon juice

1 tablespoon water

Salt and pepper to taste

Fresh cilantro for garnish (optional)

NUTRITIONAL VALUE

400 calories,

15g protein,

18g fat,

50g carbohydrates,

12g fiber.

DIRECTIONS

1.1. Arrange cooked quinoa or brown rice, cooked chickpeas, shredded purple cabbage, sliced bell peppers, shredded carrots, cherry tomatoes, and sliced avocado in a bowl.

2.2. In a small bowl, whisk together tahini, lemon juice, water, salt, and pepper to make the dressing.

3.3. Drizzle the dressing over the Buddha bowl.

4.4. Garnish with fresh cilantro if desired, and serve immediately.

DESCRIPTION

This vibrant and nutritious Buddha bowl is filled with an array of colorful vegetables, protein-rich chickpeas, creamy avocado, and a tangy tahini dressing, creating a balanced and satisfying meal.

Thai Peanut Tofu Wrap

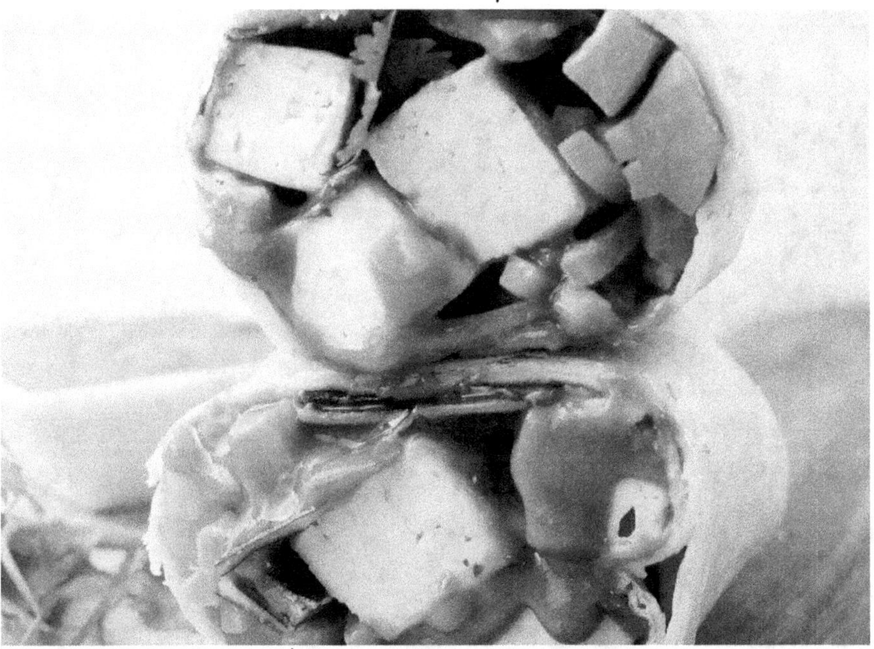

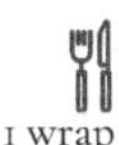 

1 wrap   20 minutes

INGREDIENTS

4 oz extra firm tofu, pressed and sliced

1 tablespoon soy sauce

1 tablespoon sesame oil

1/4 cup shredded carrots

1/4 cup sliced cucumber

1/4 cup shredded purple cabbage

2 tablespoons chopped fresh cilantro

1 tablespoon creamy peanut butter

1 tablespoon soy sauce

1 tablespoon rice vinegar

1 teaspoon maple syrup or honey

1/2 teaspoon sriracha (optional)

1 large whole wheat or spinach tortilla

NUTRITIONAL VALUE

350 calories,

15g protein,

15g fat,

40g carbohydrates,

8g fiber.

DIRECTIONS

1. 1. In a bowl, marinate sliced tofu in soy sauce and sesame oil for 10 minutes.

2. 2. Heat a skillet over medium heat and cook tofu until crispy, about 3-4 minutes per side.

3. 3. In a separate bowl, whisk together peanut butter, soy sauce, rice vinegar, maple syrup or honey, and sriracha (if using) to make the sauce.

4. 4. Spread sauce evenly over the tortilla.

5. 5. Layer cooked tofu, shredded carrots, sliced cucumber, shredded purple cabbage

6.

7. , and chopped cilantro on top of the sauce.

8. 6. Roll up the tortilla tightly, folding in the sides as you go.

9. 7. Slice the wrap in half diagonally and serve immediately, or wrap tightly in foil for later.

DESCRIPTION

This flavorful and protein-packed wrap features crispy tofu, crunchy vegetables, and a creamy Thai peanut sauce, creating a delicious and satisfying lunch option.

Butternut Squash and Kale Salad

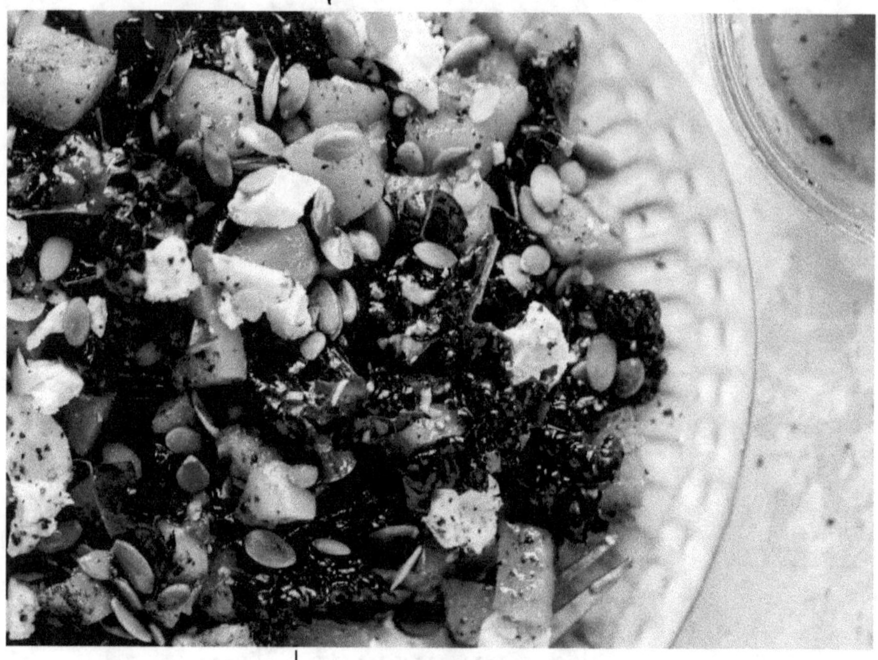

2 servings   **30 minutes**

INGREDIENTS

2 cups cubed butternut squash

2 tablespoons olive oil

Salt and pepper to taste

4 cups chopped kale

1 tablespoon olive oil

1 tablespoon balsamic vinegar

1 teaspoon maple syrup

1/4 cup toasted pepitas (pumpkin seeds)

1/4 cup crumbled goat cheese

NUTRITIONAL VALUE

250 calories,

8g protein,

12g fat,

30g carbohydrates,

5g fiber.

DIRECTIONS

1. 1. Preheat the oven to 400°F (200°C). Toss cubed butternut squash with olive oil, salt, and pepper, and spread in a single layer on a baking sheet.

2. 2. Roast squash in the preheated oven for 20-25 minutes, or until tender and caramelized.

3. 3. In a large bowl, massage chopped kale with olive oil, balsamic vinegar, maple syrup, salt, and pepper until kale is softened.

4. 4. Divide massaged kale between serving plates and top with roasted butternut squash, toasted pepitas, and crumbled goat cheese.

5. 5. Serve immediately and enjoy!

DESCRIPTION

This hearty and nutritious salad features roasted butternut squash, massaged kale, crunchy pepitas, tangy goat cheese, and a maple balsamic vinaigrette, creating a flavorful and satisfying lunch option.

Chickpea and Vegetable Curry

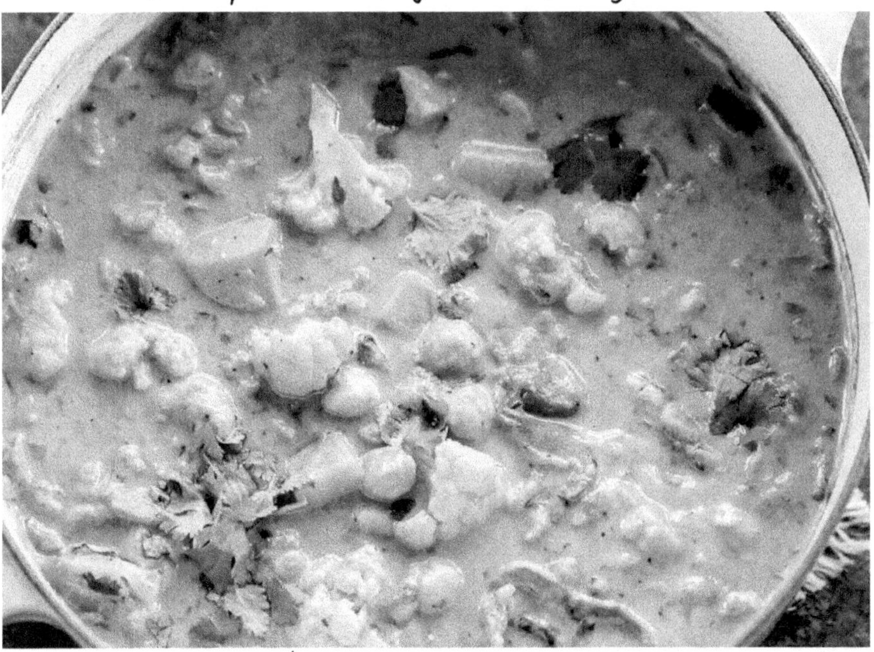

2 servings   20 minutes

INGREDIENTS

1 tablespoon coconut oil

1/2 onion, diced

2 cloves garlic, minced

1 tablespoon grated ginger

1 tablespoon curry powder

1 teaspoon ground turmeric

1/2 teaspoon ground cumin

1/2 teaspoon ground coriander

1 can (15 oz) chickpeas, drained and rinsed

1 can (14 oz) diced tomatoes

1 cup coconut milk

2 cups chopped vegetables (such as bell peppers, carrots, and cauliflower)

Salt and pepper to taste

Fresh cilantro for garnish (optional)

NUTRITIONAL VALUE

300calories,

10g protein,

15g fat,

35g carbohydrates,

8g fiber.

DIRECTIONS

1. 1. Heat coconut oil in a large skillet or pot over medium heat.
2. 2. Add diced onion, minced garlic, and grated ginger, and cook until softened, about 5 minutes.
3. 3. Stir in curry powder, turmeric, cumin, and coriander, and cook for another minute until fragrant.
4. 4. Add chickpeas, diced tomatoes, coconut milk, chopped vegetables, salt, and pepper to the skillet or pot.
5. 5. Bring the mixture to a simmer, then reduce heat to low and cook for 20-25 minutes, or until vegetables are tender and flavors have melded.
6. 6. Taste and adjust seasoning as needed.
7. 7. Serve the curry hot, garnished with fresh cilantro if desired, and accompanied by cooked rice or naan bread.

DESCRIPTION

This comforting and flavorful curry is filled with protein-rich chickpeas, colorful vegetables, and aromatic spices, making it a satisfying and nourishing meal for lunchtime.

Greek Chicken Pita Pocket

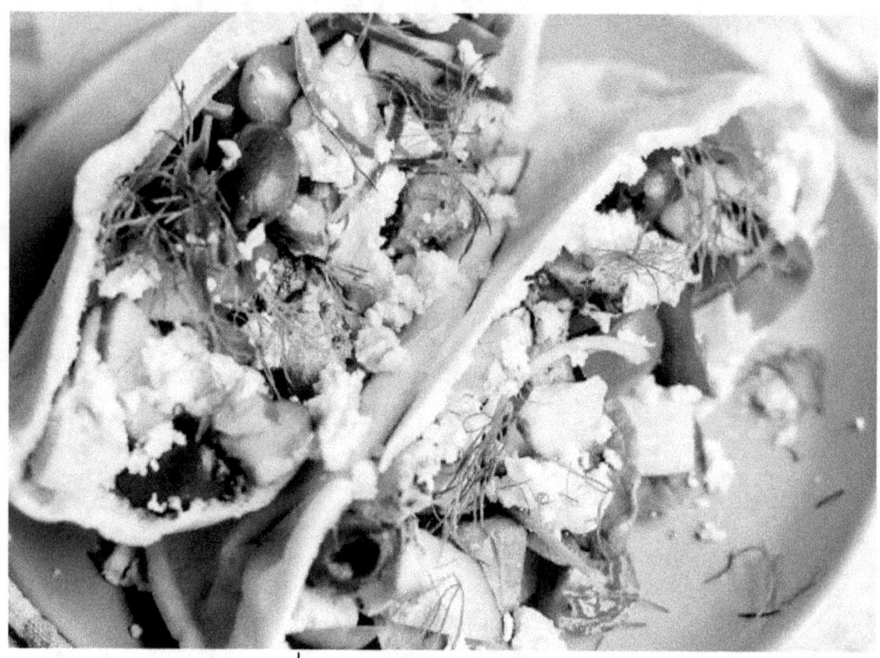

🍴 1 pita pocket   🕐 30 minutes

INGREDIENTS

1 boneless, skinless chicken breast

1 tablespoon olive oil

1 teaspoon dried oregano

Salt and pepper to taste

1 whole wheat pita pocket

2 tablespoons tzatziki sauce

1/4 cup sliced cucumber

1/4 cup diced tomatoes

2 tablespoons crumbled feta cheese

Fresh parsley for garnish (optional)

NUTRITIONAL VALUE

350 calories,

25g protein,

10g fat,

35g carbohydrates,

6g fiber.

DIRECTIONS

1.1. Preheat the grill or grill pan over medium-high heat.

2.2. Season chicken breast with olive oil, dried oregano, salt, and pepper.

3.3. Grill chicken breast for 5-6 minutes per side, or until cooked through and no longer pink in the center.

4.4. Let chicken rest for a few minutes, then slice into strips.

5.5. Warm pita pocket in the microwave or on the grill.

6.6. Spread tzatziki sauce inside the pita pocket.

7.7. Fill the pita pocket with grilled chicken strips, sliced cucumber, diced tomatoes, and crumbled feta cheese.

8.8. Garnish with fresh parsley if desired, and serve immediately.

DESCRIPTION

This delicious and protein-packed pita pocket is filled with grilled chicken, crisp vegetables, tangy tzatziki sauce, and crumbled feta cheese, creating a satisfying and flavorful lunch option.

Minestrone Soup

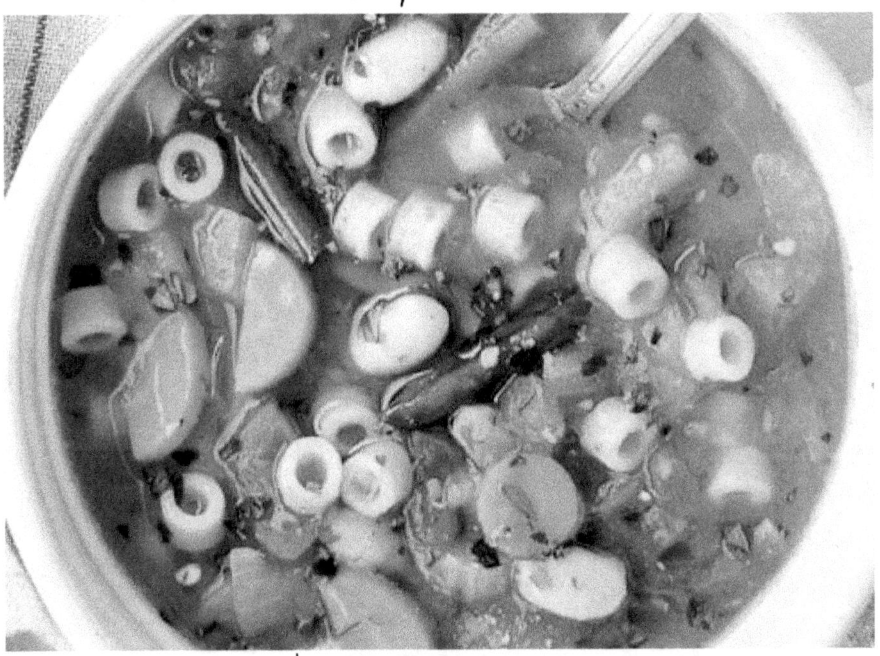

2 servings   40 minutes

INGREDIENTS

1 tablespoon olive oil

1/2 onion, diced

2 cloves garlic, minced

2 carrots, diced

2 celery stalks, diced

1 can (15 oz) diced tomatoes

4 cups vegetable broth

1 can (15 oz) cannellini beans, drained and rinsed

1/2 cup small pasta (such as ditalini or macaroni)

1 teaspoon dried thyme

1 teaspoon dried oregano

Salt and pepper to taste

Grated Parmesan cheese for serving (optional)

NUTRITIONAL VALUE

250 calories,

10g protein,

5g fat,

40g carbohydrates,

8g fiber.

DIRECTIONS

1.1. Heat olive oil in a large pot over medium heat.

2.2. Add diced onion and minced garlic, and cook until softened, about 5 minutes.

3.3. Add diced carrots and celery, and cook for another 5 minutes.

4.4. Stir in diced tomatoes, vegetable broth, cannellini beans, small pasta, dried thyme, dried oregano, salt, and pepper.

5.5. Bring the soup to a boil, then reduce heat to low and simmer for 20-25 minutes, or until vegetables are tender and pasta is cooked.

6.6. Taste and adjust seasoning as needed.

7.7. Ladle the soup into bowls, garnish with grated Parmesan cheese if desired, and serve hot.

DESCRIPTION

This classic Italian soup is loaded with vegetables, beans, pasta, and aromatic herbs, creating a hearty and satisfying meal-in-a-bowl for lunchtime.

BBQ Chickpea Salad Bowl

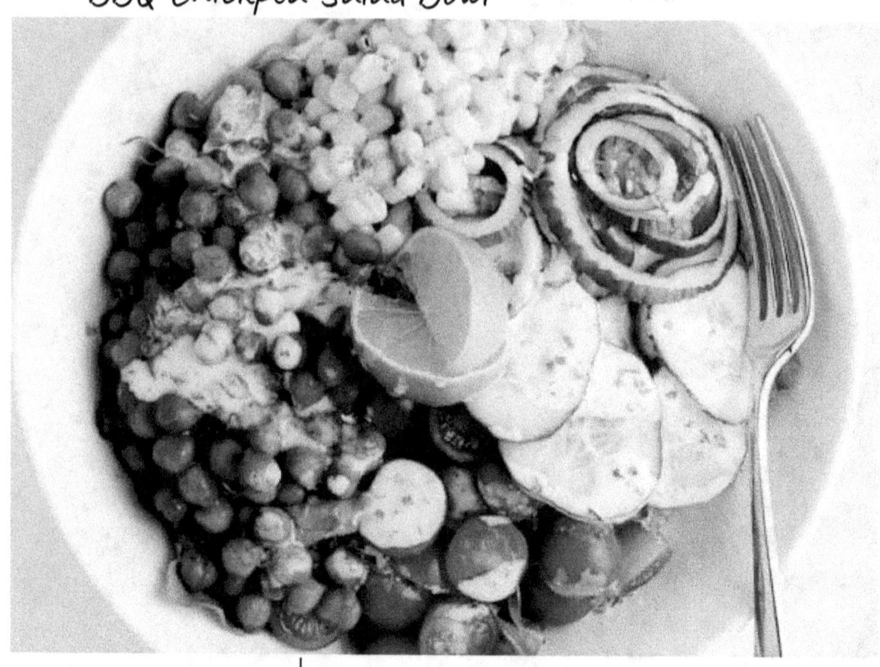

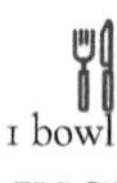
1 bowl

30 minutes

INGREDIENTS

1 can (15 oz) chickpeas, drained and rinsed

1 tablespoon olive oil

1 teaspoon smoked paprika

1/2 teaspoon garlic powder

1/2 teaspoon onion powder

Salt and pepper to taste

2 cups mixed salad greens

1/2 cup cherry tomatoes, halved

1/4 cup diced red onion

1/4 cup corn kernels (fresh or thawed frozen)

1/2 avocado, sliced

2 tablespoons barbecue sauce

NUTRITIONAL VALUE

300 calories,

10g protein,

15g fat,

35g carbohydrates,

8g fiber.

DIRECTIONS

1.1. Preheat the oven to 400°F (200°C). Toss chickpeas with olive oil, smoked paprika, garlic powder, onion powder, salt, and pepper, and spread in a single layer on a baking sheet.

2.2. Roast chickpeas in the preheated oven for 20-25 minutes, or until crispy and golden brown.

3.3. In a bowl, assemble mixed salad greens, cherry tomatoes, diced red onion, corn kernels, sliced avocado, and roasted chickpeas.

4.4. Drizzle barbecue sauce over the salad bowl.

5.5. Toss gently to combine, and serve immediately.

DESCRIPTION

This BBQ chickpea salad bowl features smoky roasted chickpeas, crisp vegetables, creamy avocado, and tangy barbecue sauce, creating a delicious and satisfying lunch option.

Nourishing Dinners
Flavorful Fish and Seafood Dishes
Plant-Powered Main Courses
Comforting Grain and Pasta Recipes

Lemon Garlic Baked Salmon

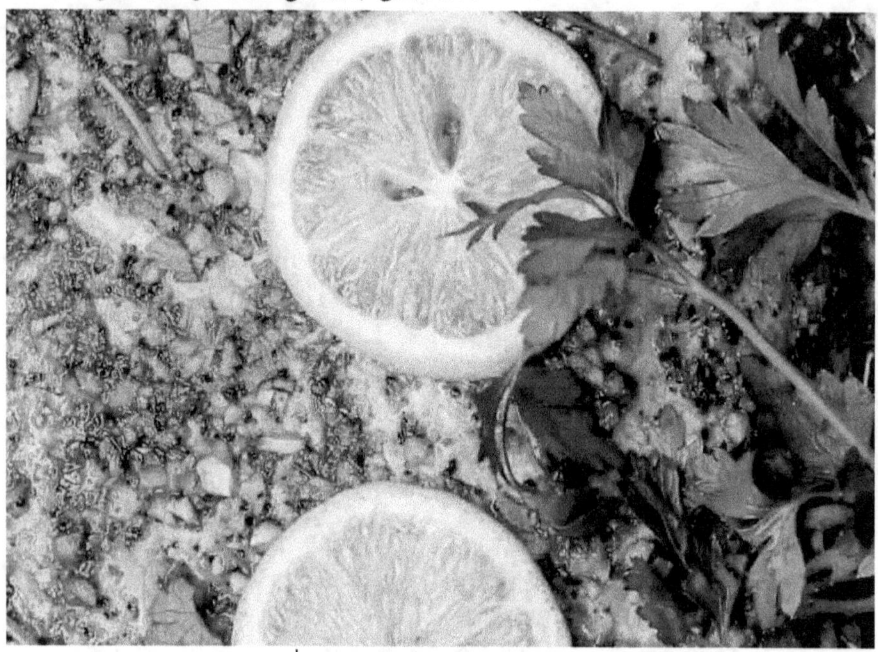

2 serving   30 minutes

INGREDIENTS

2 salmon fillets

2 tablespoons olive oil

2 cloves garlic, minced

Zest of 1 lemon

Juice of 1 lemon

1 teaspoon dried oregano

Salt and pepper to taste

Fresh parsley for garnish (optional)

NUTRITIONAL VALUE

300 calories,

25g protein,

15g fat,

5g carbohydrates,

1g fiber.

DIRECTIONS

1.1. Preheat the oven to 375°F (190°C). Place salmon fillets on a baking sheet lined with parchment paper.

2.2. In a small bowl, whisk together olive oil, minced garlic, lemon zest, lemon juice, dried oregano, salt, and pepper.

3.3. Pour the marinade over the salmon fillets, ensuring they are evenly coated.

4.4. Bake in the preheated oven for 15-20 minutes, or until salmon is cooked through and flakes easily with a fork.

5.5. Garnish with fresh parsley if desired, and serve hot.

DESCRIPTION

This flavorful baked salmon is marinated in a zesty lemon garlic sauce and baked to perfection, creating a delicious and healthy dinner option.

Chickpea and Vegetable Stir-Fry

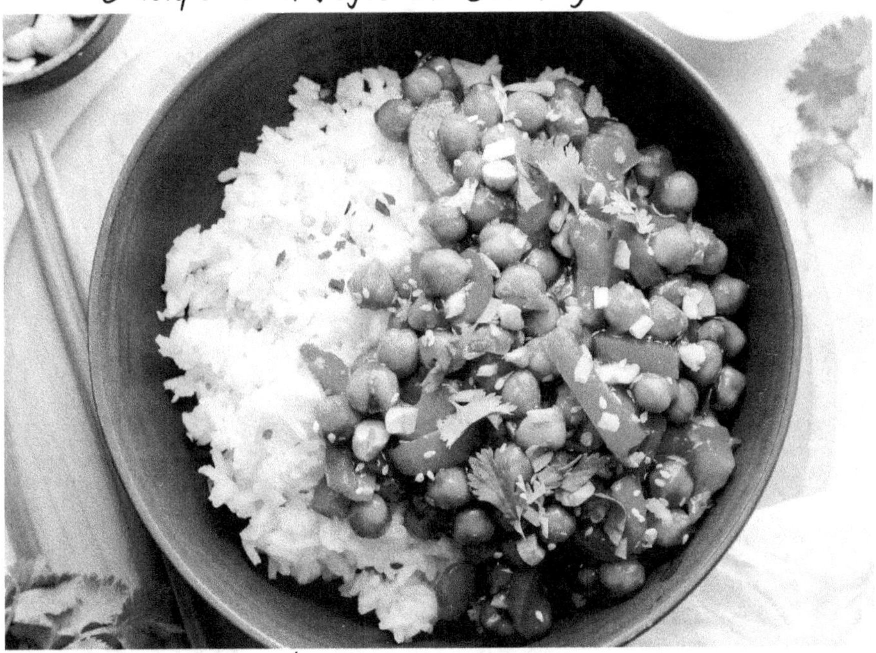

2 serving   20 minutes

INGREDIENTS

1 tablespoon sesame oil

1/2 onion, sliced

2 cloves garlic, minced

1 bell pepper, sliced

1 cup broccoli florets

1 can (15 oz) chickpeas, drained and rinsed

2 tablespoons soy sauce

1 tablespoon rice vinegar

1 teaspoon sesame seeds for garnish (optional)

Cooked rice or quinoa for serving

NUTRITIONAL VALUE

300 calories,

10g protein,

10g fat,

40g carbohydrates,

10g fiber.

DIRECTIONS

1.1. Heat sesame oil in a large skillet or wok over medium heat.

2.2. Add sliced onion and minced garlic, and cook until softened, about 2-3 minutes.

3.3. Add sliced bell pepper and broccoli florets to the skillet, and cook for another 5 minutes, or until vegetables are tender-crisp.

4.4. Stir in chickpeas, soy sauce, and rice vinegar, and cook for another 2-3 minutes, or until heated through.

5.5. Serve stir-fry over cooked rice or quinoa, garnished with sesame seeds if desired.

DESCRIPTION

This flavorful stir-fry features protein-packed chickpeas, colorful vegetables, and a savory sauce, creating a satisfying plant-powered main course.

Creamy Mushroom and Spinach Pasta

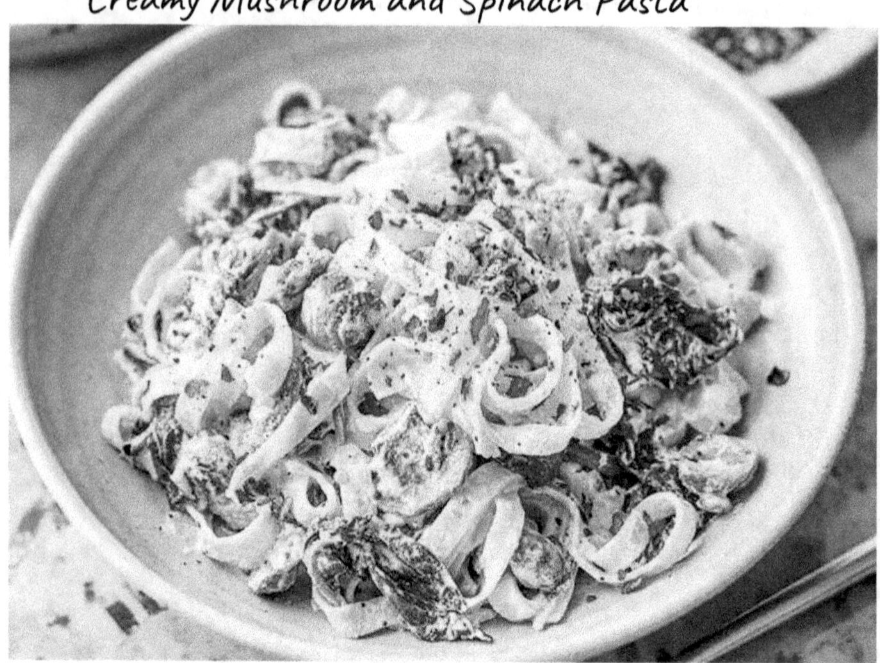

🍴 **2 serving**   🕐 **30 minutes**

INGREDIENTS

8 oz pasta (such as fettuccine or
linguine)

2 tablespoons olive oil

8 oz cremini mushrooms, sliced

2 cloves garlic, minced

2 cups baby spinach

1 cup heavy cream

1/4 cup grated Parmesan cheese

Salt and pepper to taste

Fresh parsley for garnish (optional)

NUTRITIONAL VALUE

400 calories,

10g protein,

20g fat,

45g carbohydrates,

3g fiber.

DIRECTIONS

1. 1. Cook pasta according to package instructions until al dente. Drain and set aside.
2. 2. Heat olive oil in a large skillet over medium heat.
3. 3. Add sliced mushrooms and minced garlic to the skillet, and cook until mushrooms are golden brown and tender, about 5-7 minutes.
4. 4. Stir in baby spinach and cook until wilted, about 2-3 minutes.
5. 5. Pour heavy cream into the skillet and bring to a simmer. Cook for 3-4 minutes, or until the sauce thickens slightly.
6. 6. Stir in grated Parmesan cheese until melted and smooth.
7. 7. Season with salt and pepper to taste.
8. 8. Add cooked pasta to the skillet and toss until well coated in the sauce.
9. 9. Serve pasta hot, garnished with fresh parsley if desired.

DESCRIPTION

This comforting pasta dish features
creamy mushroom sauce, wilted
spinach, and al dente pasta,
creating a satisfying and flavorful
dinner option.

Moroccan Chickpea Tagine

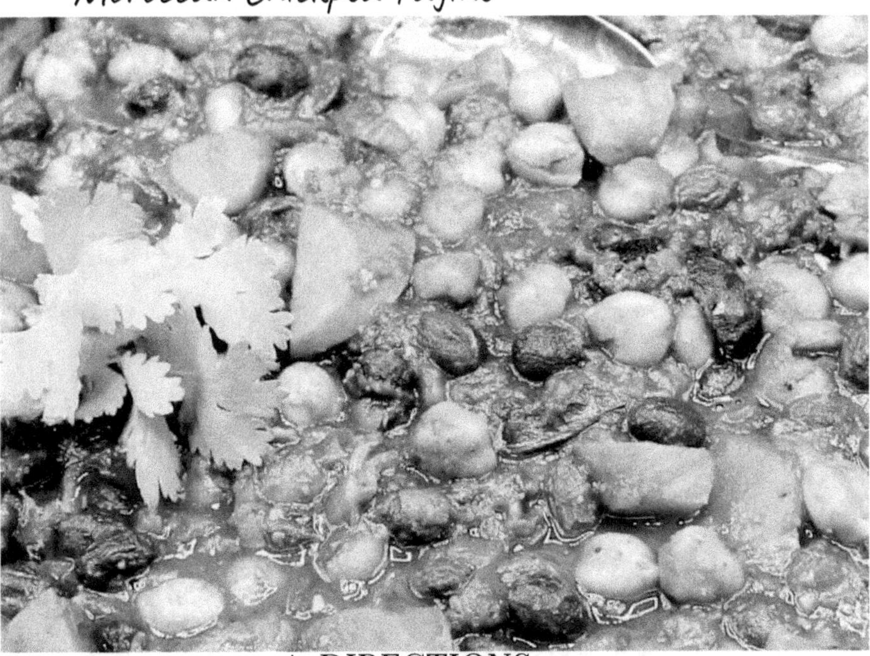

4 serving 40 minutes

INGREDIENTS

2 tablespoons olive oil

1 onion, diced

2 cloves garlic, minced

1 teaspoon ground cumin

1 teaspoon ground coriander

1/2 teaspoon ground cinnamon

1/2 teaspoon ground turmeric

1 can (15 oz) chickpeas, drained and rinsed

1 can (14 oz) diced tomatoes

1/2 cup dried apricots, chopped

1 cup vegetable broth

Salt and pepper to taste

Cooked couscous for serving

Fresh cilantro for garnish (optional)

NUTRITIONAL VALUE

350 calories,

10g protein,

10g fat,

50g carbohydrates,

8g fiber.

DIRECTIONS

1.1. Heat olive oil in a large pot over medium heat.

2.2. Add diced onion and minced garlic to the pot, and cook until softened, about 5 minutes.

3.3. Stir in ground cumin, ground coriander, ground cinnamon, and ground turmeric, and cook for another minute until fragrant.

4.4. Add drained chickpeas, diced tomatoes, chopped dried apricots, and vegetable broth to the pot. Season with salt and pepper to taste.

5.5. Bring the mixture to a boil, then reduce heat to low and simmer for 20-25 minutes, or until flavors have melded and sauce has thickened.

6.6. Taste and adjust seasoning as needed.

7.7. Serve tagine hot, over cooked couscous, garnished with fresh cilantro if desired.

DESCRIPTION

This fragrant and flavorful tagine features spiced chickpeas, sweet dried apricots, and aromatic spices, creating a hearty and comforting one-pot meal.

Baked Stuffed Bell Peppers

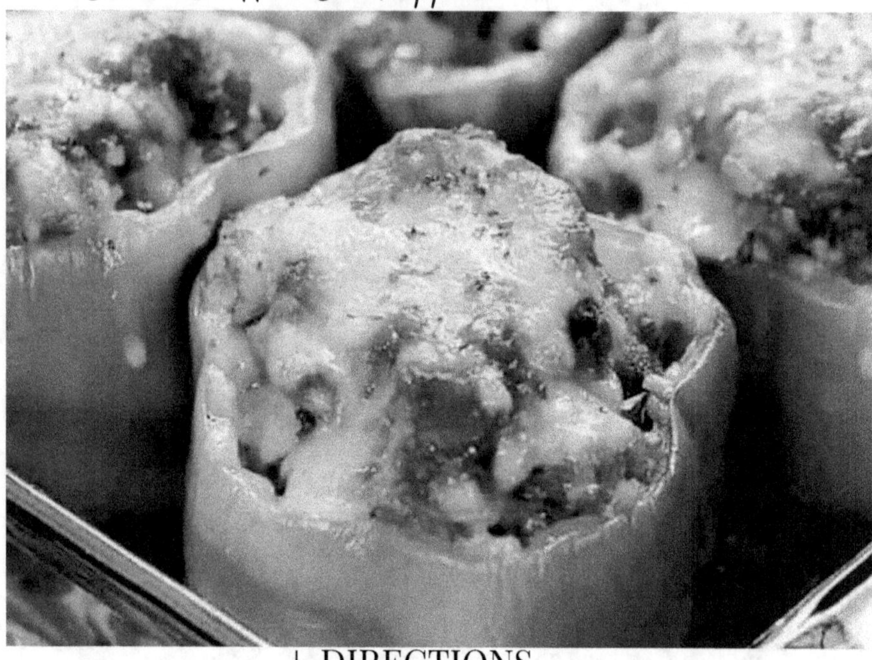

4 serving   45 minutes

INGREDIENTS

4 large bell peppers (any color)

1 cup cooked quinoa

1 can (15 oz) black beans, drained and rinsed

1 cup corn kernels (fresh or thawed frozen)

1/2 cup diced tomatoes

1/4 cup chopped fresh cilantro

1 teaspoon ground cumin

1/2 teaspoon chili powder

Salt and pepper to taste

1/2 cup shredded cheddar cheese (optional)

NUTRITIONAL VALUE

300 calories,

10g protein,

5g fat,

50g carbohydrates,

10g fiber.

DIRECTIONS

1. 1. Preheat the oven to 375°F (190°C). Cut the tops off the bell peppers and remove the seeds and membranes.
2. 2. In a large bowl, combine cooked quinoa, black beans, corn kernels, diced tomatoes, chopped cilantro, ground cumin, chili powder, salt, and pepper.
3. 3. Stuff the mixture into the bell peppers, pressing down gently to pack it in.
4. 4. Place stuffed bell peppers in a baking dish, standing upright.
5. 5. Cover the baking dish with aluminum foil and bake in the preheated oven for 30-35 minutes, or until bell peppers are tender.
6. 6. If using shredded cheddar cheese, remove the foil from the baking dish and sprinkle cheese over the tops of the stuffed bell peppers. Return to the oven and bake for an additional 5 minutes, or until cheese is melted and bubbly.
7. 7. Serve stuffed bell peppers hot, garnished with additional chopped cilantro if desired.

DESCRIPTION

This BBQ chickpea salad bowl features smoky roasted chickpeas, crisp vegetables, creamy avocado, and tangy barbecue sauce, creating a delicious and satisfying lunch option.

Teriyaki Tofu Stir-Fry

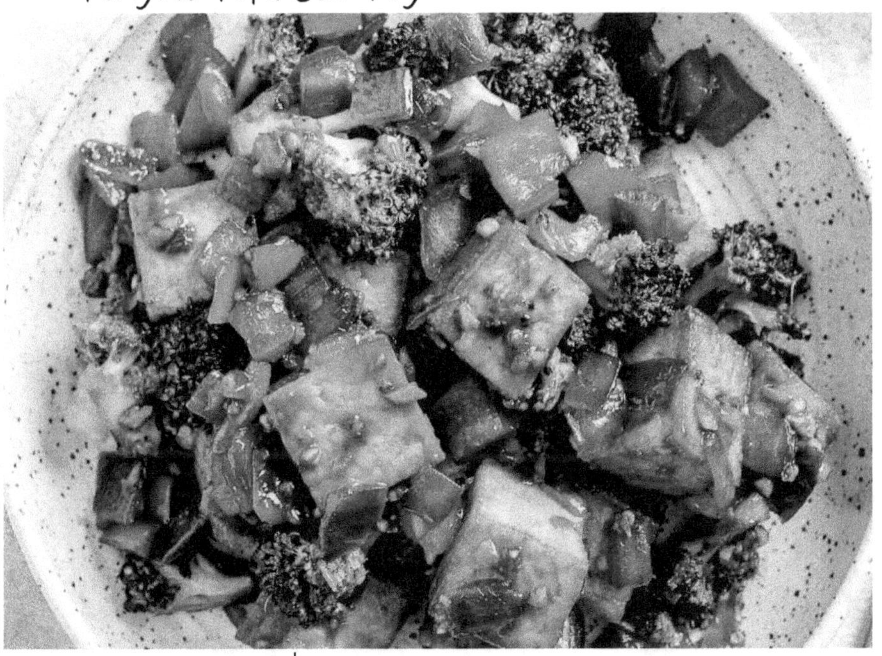

2 serving   30 minutes

INGREDIENTS

8 oz extra firm tofu, pressed and cubed

2 tablespoons cornstarch

2 tablespoons soy sauce

1 tablespoon sesame oil

1 tablespoon olive oil

1/2 onion, sliced

1 bell pepper, sliced

1 cup broccoli florets

1/4 cup teriyaki sauce

Cooked rice for serving

Sliced green onions for garnish (optional)

NUTRITIONAL VALUE

350 calories,

15g protein,

15g fat,

40g carbohydrates,

5g fiber.

DIRECTIONS

1.1. Toss cubed tofu in cornstarch until coated.

2.2. In a skillet, heat sesame oil over medium heat. Add tofu cubes and cook until crispy and golden brown on all sides, about 5-7 minutes. Remove tofu from skillet and set aside.

3.3. In the same skillet, heat olive oil over medium heat. Add sliced onion, bell pepper, and broccoli florets, and cook until vegetables are tender-crisp, about 5 minutes.

4.4. Return crispy tofu to the skillet and pour teriyaki sauce over the mixture. Stir to coat evenly and cook for another 2-3 minutes.

5.5. Serve stir-fry hot, over cooked rice, garnished with sliced green onions if desired.

DESCRIPTION

This flavorful stir-fry features crispy tofu, colorful vegetables, and a sweet and savory teriyaki sauce, creating a delicious and satisfying plant-powered main course.

Creamy Tomato Basil Pasta

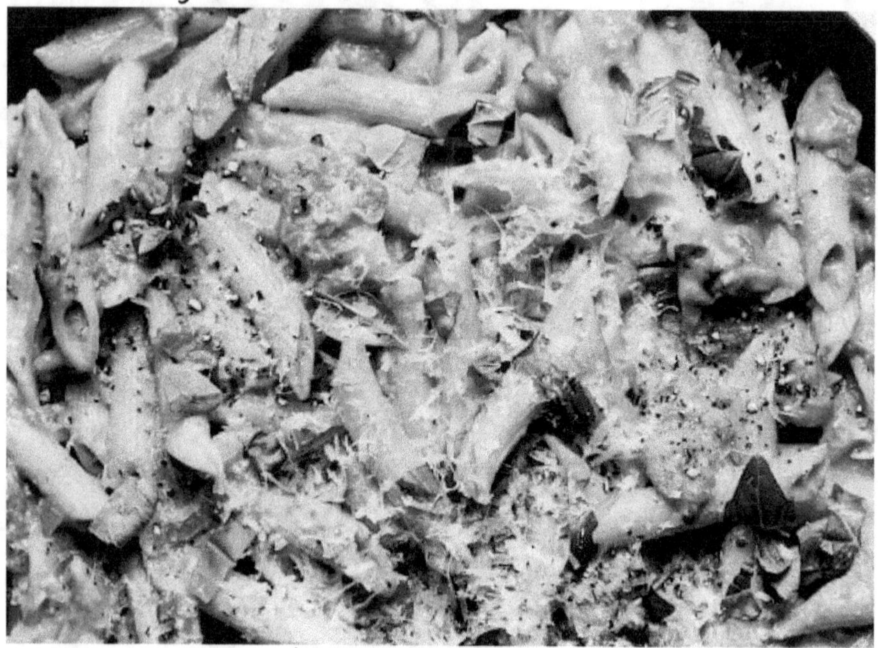

2 serving   30 minutes

INGREDIENTS

8 oz pasta (such as penne or spaghetti)

2 tablespoons olive oil

2 cloves garlic, minced

1 can (14 oz) diced tomatoes

1/2 cup heavy cream

1/4 cup grated Parmesan cheese

1/4 cup chopped fresh basil leaves

Salt and pepper to taste

NUTRITIONAL VALUE

400 calories,

10g protein,

20g fat,

45g carbohydrates,

3g fiber.

DIRECTIONS

1.1. Cook pasta according to package instructions until al dente. Drain and set aside.

2.2. In a skillet, heat olive oil over medium heat. Add minced garlic and cook until fragrant, about 1 minute.

3.3. Stir in diced tomatoes and cook for another 5 minutes, allowing the flavors to meld.

4.4. Reduce heat to low and pour heavy cream into the skillet. Stir to combine and simmer for 3-4 minutes.

5.5. Stir in grated Parmesan cheese until melted and smooth.

6.6. Season with salt and pepper to taste.

7.7. Add cooked pasta to the skillet and toss until well coated in the sauce.

8.8. Serve pasta hot, garnished with chopped fresh basil leaves.

DESCRIPTION

This comforting pasta dish features a creamy tomato basil sauce, al dente pasta, and fresh basil leaves, creating a satisfying and flavorful dinner option.

Lentil and Vegetable Curry

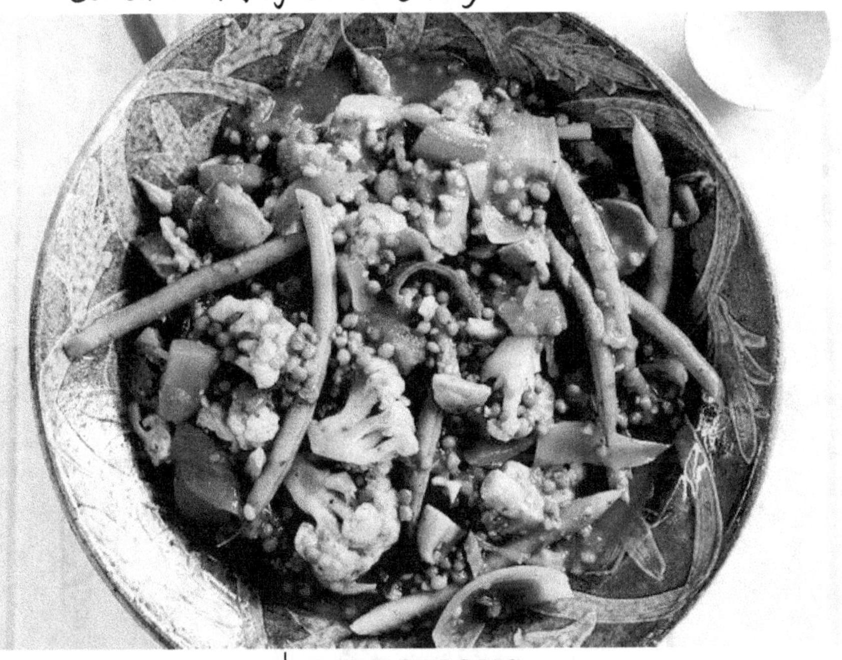

4 serving 40 minutes

INGREDIENTS

1 tablespoon coconut oil

1/2 onion, diced

2 cloves garlic, minced

1 tablespoon grated ginger

1 tablespoon curry powder

1/2 teaspoon ground turmeric

1/2 teaspoon ground cumin

1/2 teaspoon ground coriander

1 cup dried green or brown lentils, rinsed

4 cups vegetable broth

1 can (14 oz) diced tomatoes

2 cups chopped vegetables (such as carrots, bell peppers, and zucchini)

Salt and pepper to taste

Fresh cilantro for garnish (optional)

Cooked rice or naan bread for serving

NUTRITIONAL VALUE

300 calories,

15g protein,

5g fat,

50g carbohydrates,

10g fiber.

DIRECTIONS

1. 1. Heat coconut oil in a large pot over medium heat.
2. 2. Add diced onion, minced garlic, and grated ginger to the pot, and cook until softened, about 5 minutes.
3. 3. Stir in curry powder, ground turmeric, ground cumin, and ground coriander, and cook for another minute until fragrant.
4. 4. Add rinsed lentils, vegetable broth, diced tomatoes, chopped vegetables, salt, and pepper to the pot.
5. 5. Bring the mixture to a boil, then reduce heat to low and simmer for 20-25 minutes, or until lentils are tender and vegetables are cooked.
6. 6. Taste and adjust seasoning as needed.
7. 7. Serve curry hot, over cooked rice or with naan bread, garnished with fresh cilantro if desired.

DESCRIPTION

This hearty and flavorful curry features protein-rich lentils, colorful vegetables, and aromatic spices, creating a satisfying and nourishing dinner option.

Lemon Garlic Shrimp Pasta

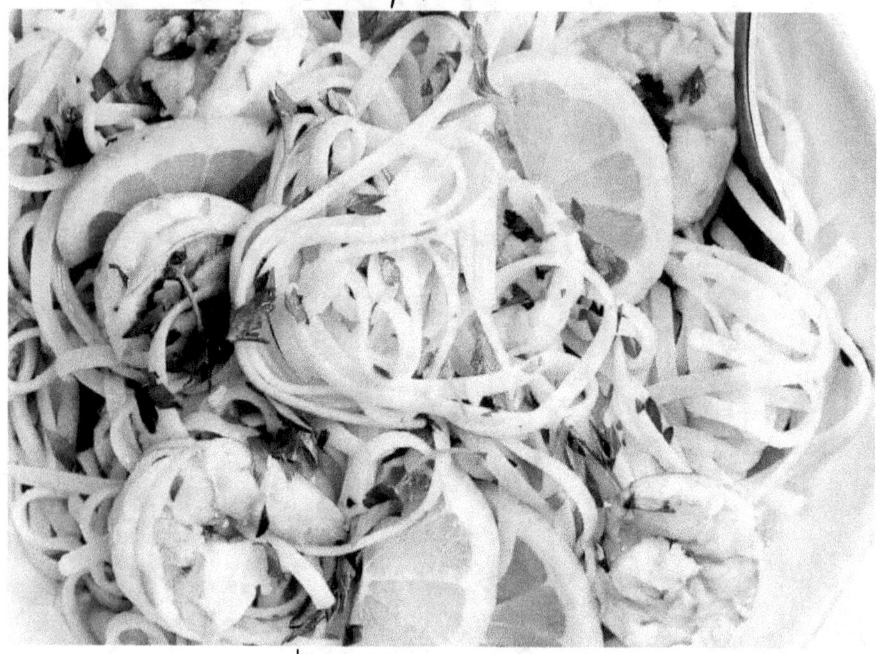

🍴 2 serving   🕐 20 minutes

INGREDIENTS

8 oz pasta (such as linguine or spaghetti)

2 tablespoons olive oil

1/2 lb large shrimp, peeled and deveined

3 cloves garlic, minced

Zest of 1 lemon

Juice of 1 lemon

1/4 cup chopped fresh parsley

Salt and pepper to taste

Grated Parmesan cheese for serving (optional)

NUTRITIONAL VALUE

350 calories,

20g protein,

15g fat,

40g carbohydrates,

3g fiber.

DIRECTIONS

1.1. Cook pasta according to package instructions until al dente. Drain and set aside.

2.2. In a skillet, heat olive oil over medium heat. Add minced garlic and cook until fragrant, about 1 minute.

3.3. Add peeled and deveined shrimp

4.

5. to the skillet, and cook until pink and opaque, about 2–3 minutes per side.

6.4. Stir in lemon zest, lemon juice, chopped fresh parsley, salt, and pepper.

7.5. Add cooked pasta to the skillet and toss until well coated in the sauce.

8.6. Serve pasta hot, with grated Parmesan cheese if desired.

DESCRIPTION

This light and refreshing pasta dish feature succulent shrimp, zesty lemon, garlic, and fresh parsley, creating a flavorful and satisfying dinner option.

Moroccan Vegetable Tagine

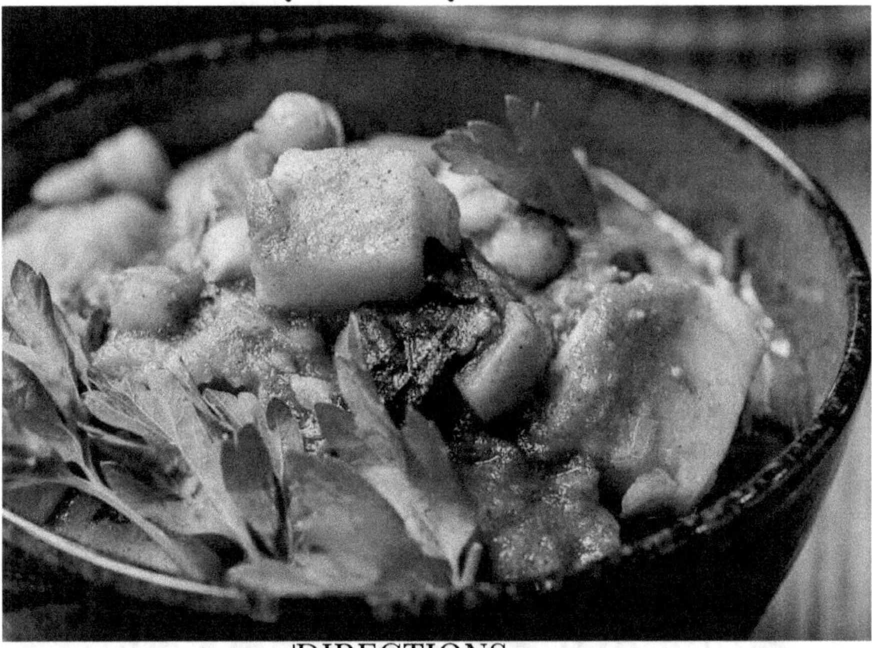

4 serving   40 minutes

INGREDIENTS

1 tablespoon olive oil

1/2 onion, diced

2 cloves garlic, minced

1 teaspoon ground cumin

1 teaspoon ground coriander

1/2 teaspoon ground cinnamon

1/2 teaspoon ground turmeric

2 carrots, diced

2 potatoes, diced

1 can (14 oz) chickpeas, drained and rinsed

1/2 cup chopped dried apricots

1/2 cup chopped dried dates

1 can (14 oz) diced tomatoes

2 cups vegetable broth

Salt and pepper to taste

Fresh cilantro for garnish (optional)

Cooked couscous for serving

NUTRITIONAL VALUE

300 calories,

10g protein,

5g fat,

50g carbohydrates,

8g fiber.

DIRECTIONS

1.1. Heat olive oil in a large pot over medium heat.

2.2. Add diced onion and minced garlic to the pot, and cook until softened, about 5 minutes.

3.3. Stir in ground cumin, ground coriander, ground cinnamon, and ground turmeric, and cook for another minute until fragrant.

4.4. Add diced carrots, diced potatoes, drained chickpeas, chopped dried apricots, chopped dried dates, diced tomatoes, and vegetable broth to the pot.

5.5. Season with salt and pepper to taste.

6.6. Bring the mixture to a boil, then reduce heat to low and simmer for 20-25 minutes, or until vegetables are tender and flavors have melded.

7.7. Taste and adjust seasoning as needed.

8.8. Serve tagine hot, over cooked couscous, garnished with fresh cilantro if desired.

DESCRIPTION

This fragrant and flavorful tagine features a medley of vegetables, aromatic spices, and sweet dried fruit, creating a hearty and comforting one-pot meal.

Trail Mix Crunch

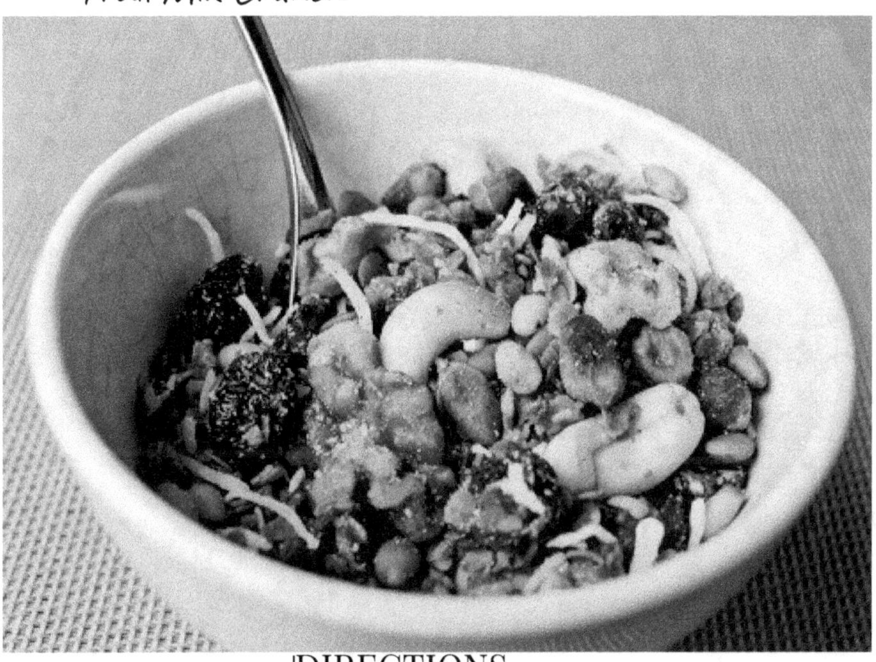

1/4 cup   5 minutes

INGREDIENTS

1/4 cup almonds

1/4 cup walnuts

2 tablespoons pumpkin seeds

2 tablespoons sunflower seeds

2 tablespoons dried cranberries

2 tablespoons raisins

NUTRITIONAL VALUE

200 calories,

5g protein,

15g fat,

15g carbohydrates,

3g fiber.

DIRECTIONS

1. 1. In a bowl, combine almonds, walnuts, pumpkin seeds, sunflower seeds, dried cranberries, and raisins.
2. 2. Mix well to combine.
3. 3. Store in an airtight container for up to one week.

DESCRIPTION

This energy-boosting mix combines nuts, seeds, and dried fruits for a satisfying snack that will keep you fueled throughout the day.

Hummus Trio Platter

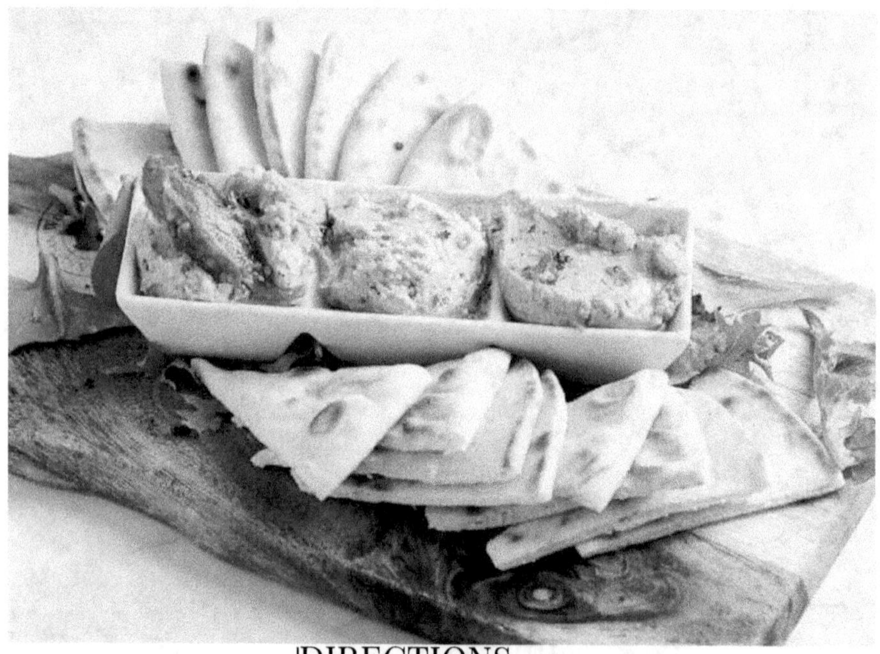

2 serving   15 minutes

INGREDIENTS

1 can (15 oz) chickpeas, drained
and rinsed
2 tablespoons tahini
2 cloves garlic, minced
Juice of 1 lemon
Salt and pepper to taste
1/2 cup roasted red peppers
1/2 cup chopped spinach
1/4 cup chopped artichoke hearts
Assorted fresh vegetables for
dipping (such as carrots,
cucumber, and bell peppers)

NUTRITIONAL VALUE

150 calories,

5g protein,

8g fat,

15g carbohydrates,

5g fiber.

DIRECTIONS

1. 1. In a food processor, combine chickpeas, tahini, minced garlic, lemon juice, salt, and pepper. Blend until smooth to make classic hummus. Transfer to a serving bowl.

2. 2. Add roasted red peppers to the food processor and blend until smooth to make roasted red pepper hummus. Transfer to a serving bowl.

3. 3. Add chopped spinach and artichoke hearts to the food processor and blend until smooth to make spinach and artichoke hummus. Transfer to a serving bowl.

4. 4. Arrange assorted fresh vegetables on a platter alongside the hummus trio.

5. 5. Serve immediately and enjoy!

DESCRIPTION

This guilt-free dip trio features classic hummus, roasted red pepper hummus, and spinach and artichoke hummus, served with fresh vegetables for dipping.

No-Bake Peanut Butter Granola Bars

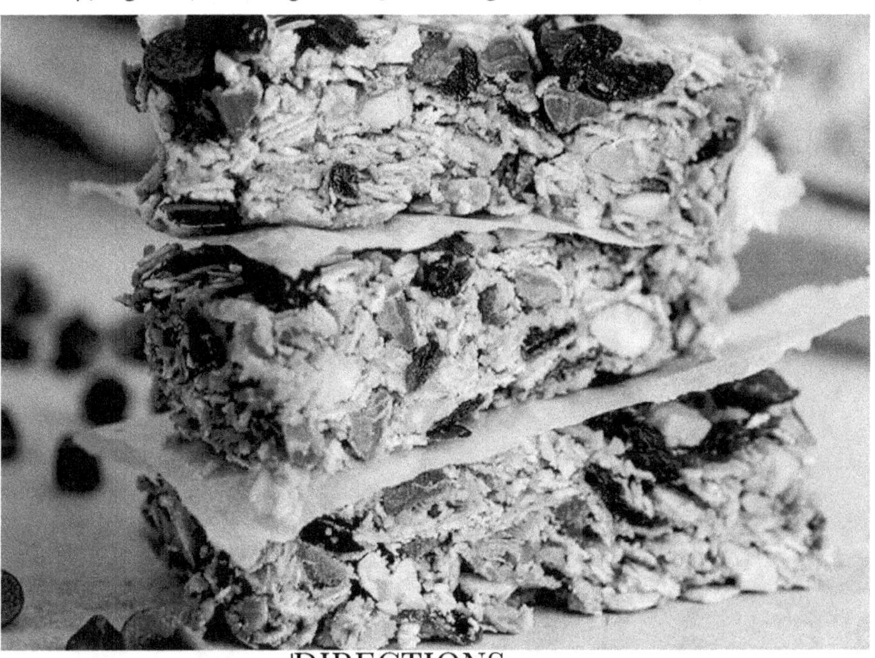

🍴 6 bars   🕐 15 minutes

INGREDIENTS

1 cup rolled oats

1/2 cup creamy peanut butter

1/4 cup honey

1/4 cup chocolate chips

1/4 teaspoon salt

NUTRITIONAL VALUE

200 calories,

5g protein,

10g fat,

20g carbohydrates,

3g fiber.

DIRECTIONS

1. 1. Line a square baking dish with parchment paper, leaving some overhang on the sides.
2. 2. In a microwave-safe bowl, combine peanut butter and honey. Microwave in 30-second intervals until melted and smooth.
3. 3. Stir in rolled oats, chocolate chips, and salt until well combined.
4. 4. Press the mixture evenly into the prepared baking dish.
5. 5. Refrigerate for at least 1 hour, or until firm.
6. 6. Lift the bars out of the dish using the parchment paper overhang and cut into squares.
7. 7. Serve and enjoy!

DESCRIPTION

These homemade granola bars are made with peanut butter, oats, honey, and chocolate chips for a delicious and satisfying snack.

Energy-Boosting Almond Butter Bites

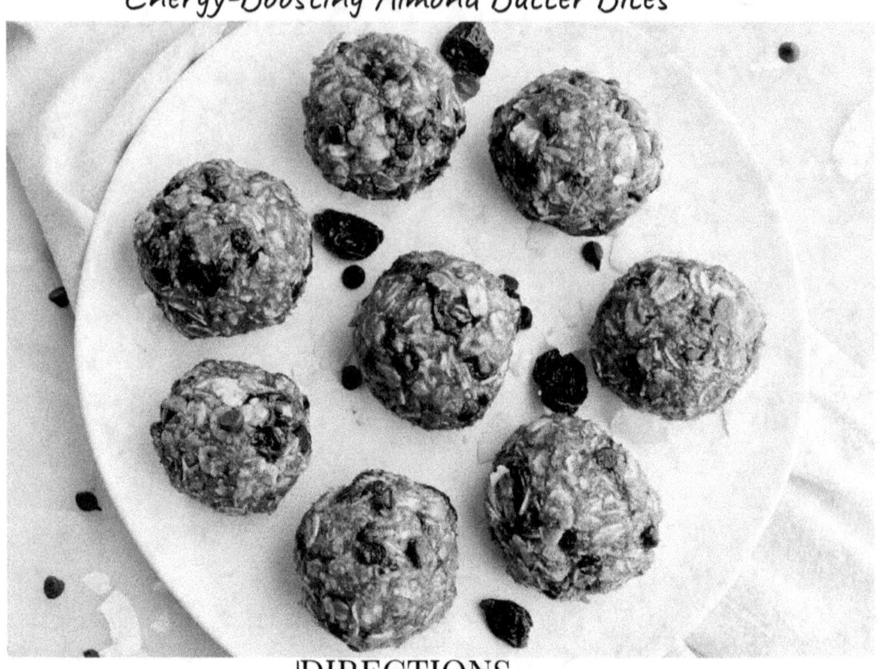

INGREDIENTS

8 bites · **20 minutes**

1/2 cup almond butter
1/2 cup pitted dates
1/4 cup rolled oats
2 tablespoons chia seeds
1/4 teaspoon vanilla extract
Pinch of salt
Shredded coconut for coating
(optional)

NUTRITIONAL VALUE

150 calories,
4g protein,
8g fat,
15g carbohydrates,
3g fiber.

DIRECTIONS

1. 1. In a food processor, combine almond butter, pitted dates, rolled oats, chia seeds, vanilla extract, and salt. Blend until a dough forms.
2. 2. Roll the dough into small balls, about 1 tablespoon each.
3. 3. If desired, roll the balls in shredded coconut to coat.
4. 4. Place the almond butter bites on a baking sheet lined with parchment paper.
5. 5. Refrigerate for at least 30 minutes, or until firm.
6. 6. Serve chilled and enjoy!

DESCRIPTION

These bite-sized treats are made with almond butter, dates, oats, and chia seeds for a nutritious and energizing snack.

Dark Chocolate Avocado Mousse

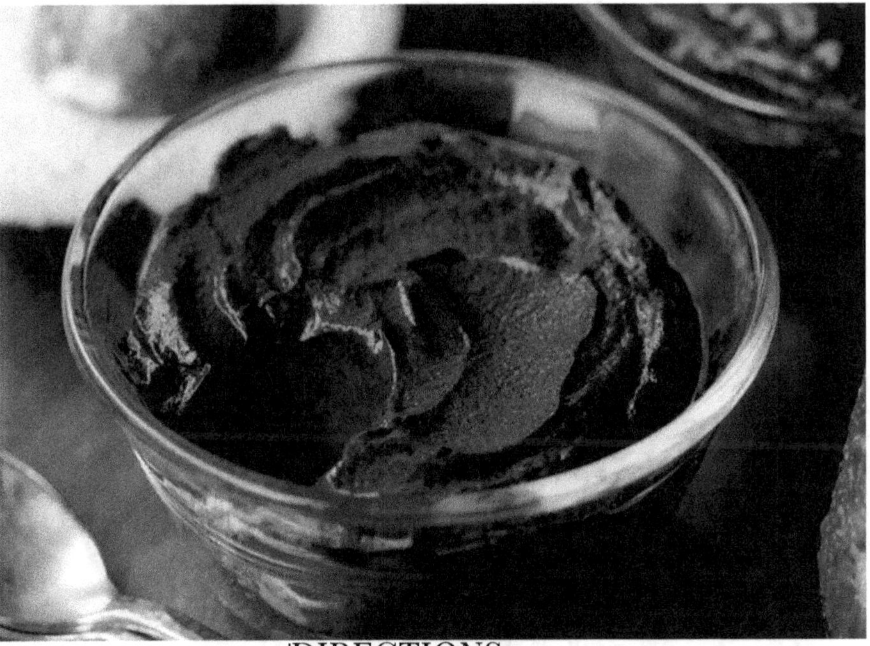

🍴 2 serving 🕐 10 minutes

INGREDIENTS

2 ripe avocados

1/4 cup cocoa powder

1/4 cup honey

1 teaspoon vanilla extract

Pinch of salt

Dark chocolate shavings for garnish (optional)

NUTRITIONAL VALUE

250 calories,

3g protein,

15g fat,

30g carbohydrates,

8g fiber.

DIRECTIONS

1.1. Cut the avocados in half and remove the pits.

2.2. Scoop the avocado flesh into a blender or food processor.

3.3. Add cocoa powder, honey, vanilla extract, and salt to the blender.

4.4. Blend until smooth and creamy, scraping down the sides as needed.

5.5. Divide the chocolate avocado mousse into serving cups.

6.6. Refrigerate for at least 30 minutes, or until chilled.

7.7. Garnish with dark chocolate shavings if desired.

8.8. Serve and enjoy!

DESCRIPTION

This decadent dessert is made with ripe avocados, cocoa powder, honey, and vanilla extract, creating a creamy and indulgent treat.

Spiced Roasted Chickpeas

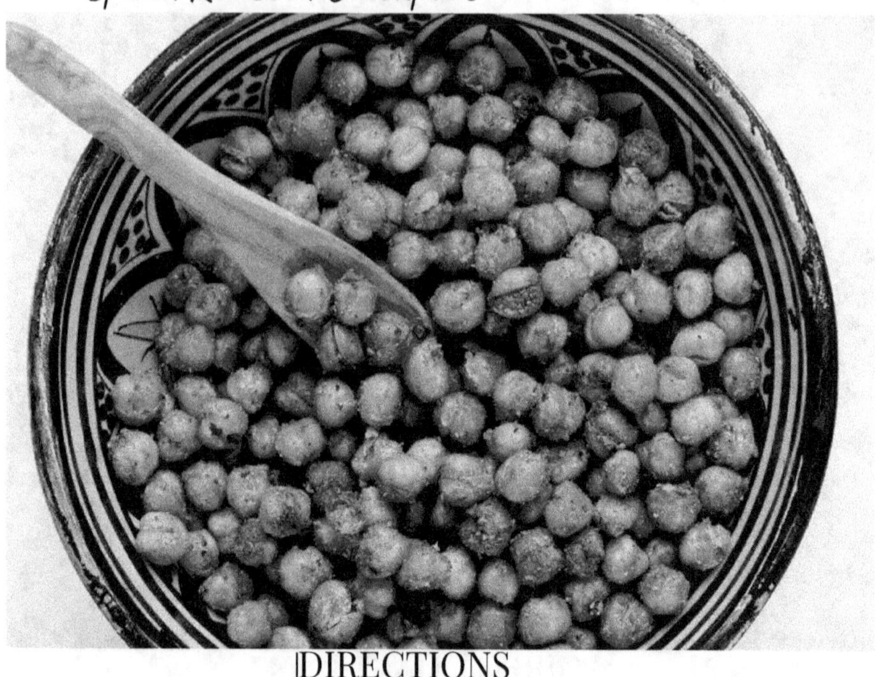

1/2 cup   **45 minutes**

INGREDIENTS

1 can (15 oz) chickpeas, drained and rinsed

1 tablespoon olive oil

1 teaspoon ground cumin

1/2 teaspoon ground coriander

1/2 teaspoon smoked paprika

1/4 teaspoon cayenne pepper

Salt to taste

NUTRITIONAL VALUE

150 calories,

5g protein,

6g fat,

20g carbohydrates,

6g fiber.

DIRECTIONS

1.1. Preheat the oven to 400°F (200°C). Line a baking sheet with parchment paper.

2.2. Pat the chickpeas dry with a paper towel and spread them out on the prepared baking sheet.

3.3. Drizzle olive oil over the chickpeas and toss to coat evenly.

4.4. In a small bowl, combine ground cumin, ground coriander, smoked paprika, cayenne pepper, and salt.

5.5. Sprinkle the spice mixture over the chickpeas and toss to coat evenly.

6.6. Roast in the preheated oven for 30-35 minutes, stirring halfway through, until golden brown and crispy.

7.7. Allow to cool slightly before serving.

8.8. Serve roasted chickpeas as a crunchy snack or salad topper.

DESCRIPTION

These crunchy roasted chickpeas are seasoned with warm spices for a flavorful and satisfying snack.

Greek Yogurt Fruit Parfait

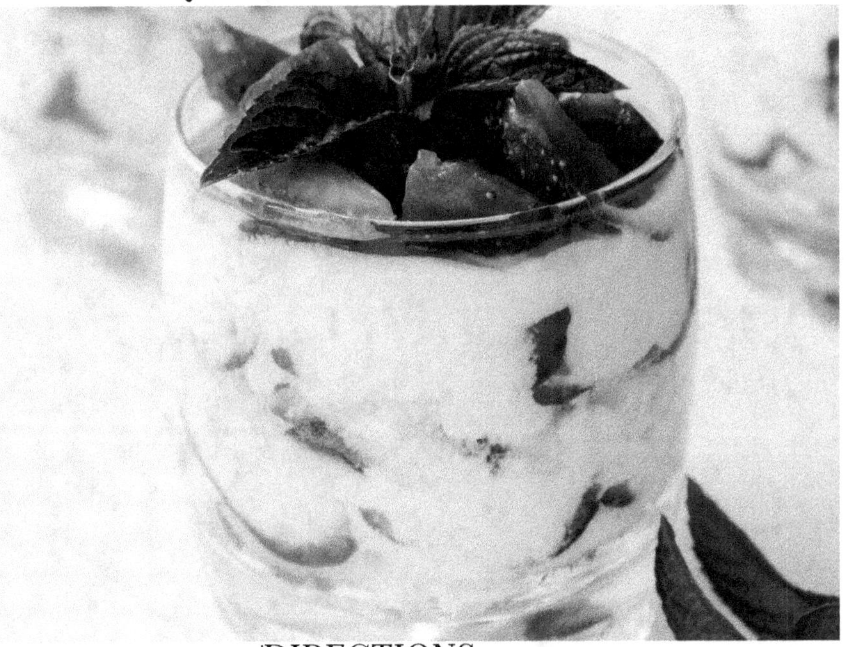

<table>
<tr><td>serving</td><td>5 minutes</td></tr>
</table>

INGREDIENTS

1/2 cup Greek yogurt

1/4 cup mixed berries (such as strawberries, blueberries, and raspberries)

1/4 cup granola

Honey for drizzling (optional)

NUTRITIONAL VALUE

200 calories,

10g protein,

5g fat,

25g carbohydrates,

3g fiber.

DIRECTIONS

1. 1. In a glass or bowl, layer Greek yogurt, mixed berries, and granola.
2. 2. Repeat the layers until the glass or bowl is filled.
3. 3. Drizzle with honey if desired.
4. 4. Serve immediately and enjoy!

DESCRIPTION

This refreshing parfait features layers of creamy Greek yogurt, fresh berries, and crunchy granola, creating a nutritious and delicious snack or dessert.

Chocolate Peanut Butter Energy Balls

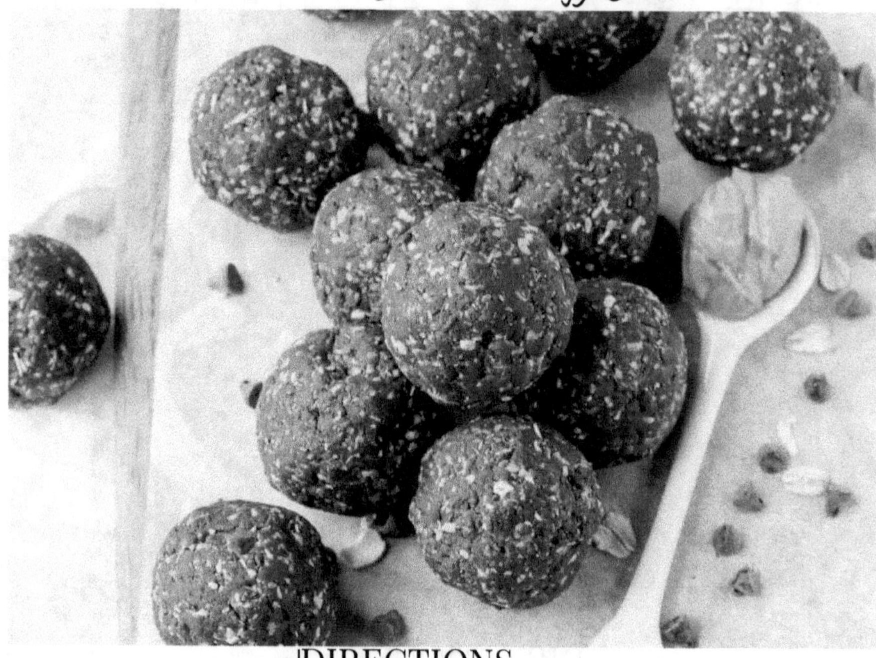

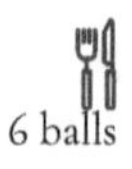 

6 balls   15 minutes

INGREDIENTS

1/2 cup rolled oats

1/4 cup creamy peanut
butter

- 2 tablespoons honey

2 tablespoons dark
chocolate chips

Pinch of salt

NUTRITIONAL VALUE

150 calories,

5g protein,

8g fat,

15g carbohydrates,

3g fiber.

DIRECTIONS

1. 1. In a bowl, combine rolled oats, creamy peanut butter, honey, dark chocolate chips, and a pinch of salt.
2. 2. Mix well until all ingredients are fully incorporated.
3. 3. Roll the mixture into small balls, about 1 tablespoon each.
4. 4. Place the energy balls on a baking sheet lined with parchment paper.
5. 5. Refrigerate for at least 30 minutes, or until firm.
6. 6. Serve chilled and enjoy!

DESCRIPTION

These no-bake energy balls are made with oats, peanut butter, honey, and dark chocolate chips for a delicious and nutritious snack on the go.

Guacamole Stuffed Mini Bell Peppers

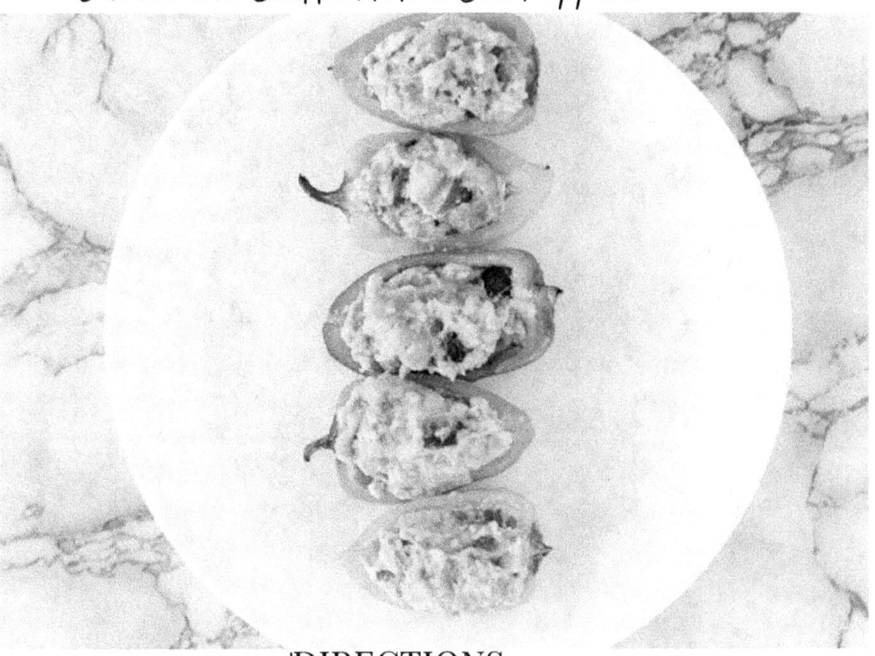

2 serving **15 minutes**

INGREDIENTS

6 mini bell peppers, halved and seeded

1 ripe avocado

1/4 cup diced tomatoes

1/4 cup diced red onion

1 tablespoon chopped cilantro

Juice of 1 lime

Salt and pepper to taste

NUTRITIONAL VALUE

100 calories,

2g protein,

8g fat,

10g carbohydrates,

4g fiber.

DIRECTIONS

1.1. In a bowl, mash the ripe avocado with a fork until smooth.

2.2. Stir in diced tomatoes, diced red onion, chopped cilantro, lime juice, salt, and pepper.

3.3. Spoon the guacamole mixture into the halved mini bell peppers.

4.4. Serve immediately and enjoy!

DESCRIPTION

These bite-sized snacks feature mini bell peppers stuffed with creamy guacamole for a flavorful and satisfying treat.

Chocolate Covered Almonds

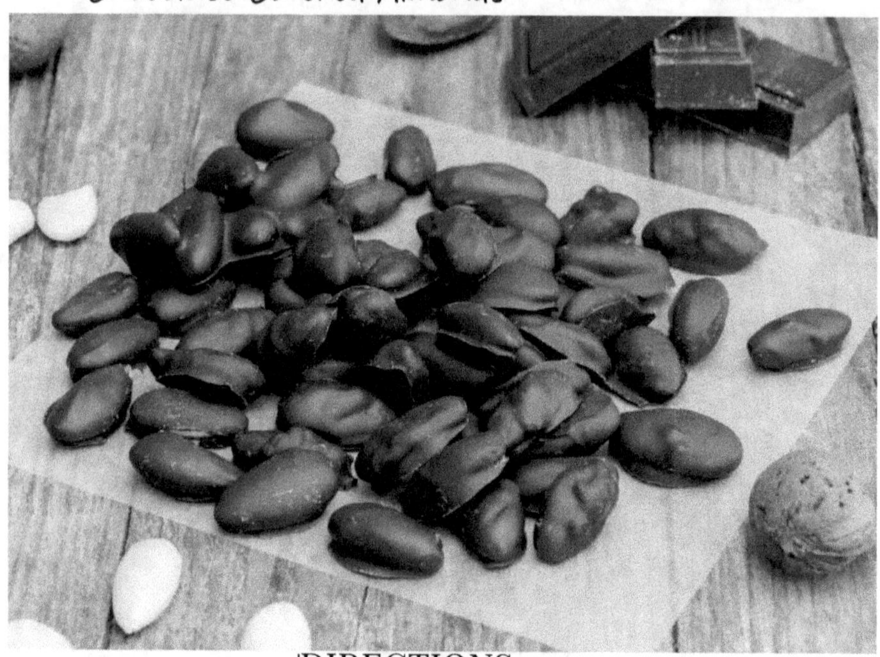

1/4 cup   **30 minutes**

INGREDIENTS

1 cup whole

almonds

4 oz dark

chocolate,

chopped

NUTRITIONAL VALUE

200 calories,

5g protein,

15g fat,

15g carbohydrates,

3g fiber.

DIRECTIONS

1.1. Line a baking sheet with parchment paper.

2.2. In a microwave-safe bowl, melt the dark chocolate in 30-second intervals, stirring in between, until smooth.

3.3. Dip each almond into the melted chocolate, coating evenly.

4.4. Place the chocolate-covered almonds on the prepared baking sheet.

5.5. Refrigerate for 20-30 minutes, or until the chocolate is set.

6.6. Serve and enjoy!

DESCRIPTION

These decadent treats feature crunchy almonds coated in rich dark chocolate for a sweet and satisfying snack.

Beverages for Brain Health
Refreshing Smoothie and
Juice Blends
Herbal Teas for Relaxation
and Focus
Infused Waters for Hydration
and Flavor
Nutrient-Rich Hot Beverage
Creations

Berry Brain Boost Smoothie

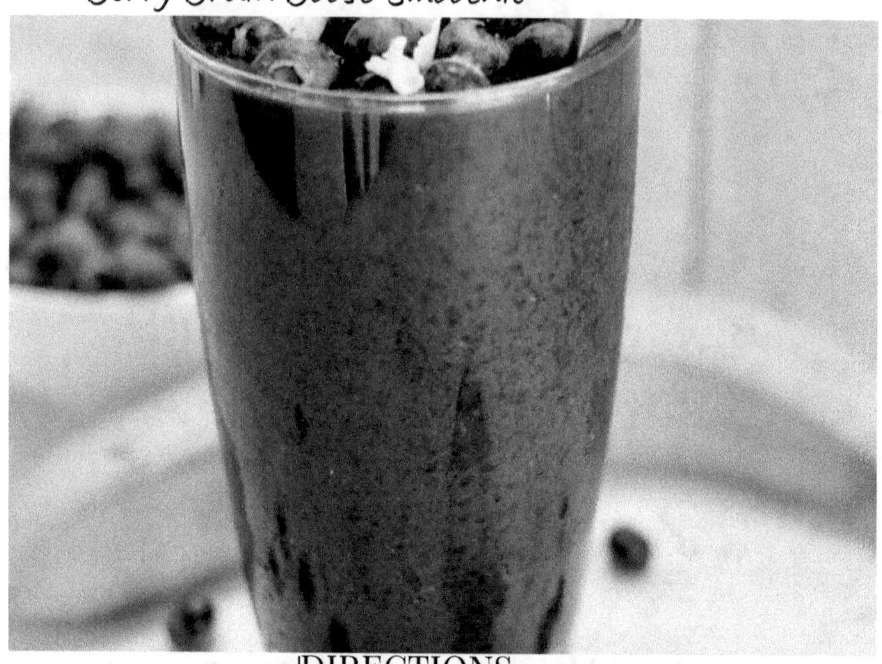

1 serving   **5 minutes**

INGREDIENTS

1/2 cup mixed berries (such as strawberries, blueberries, and raspberries)

1 banana

1 tablespoon ground flaxseeds

1/2 cup Greek yogurt

1/2 cup almond milk

Honey or maple syrup to taste (optional)

NUTRITIONAL VALUE

200 calories,

10g protein,

5g fat,

30g carbohydrates,

5g fiber.

DIRECTIONS

1. 1. Combine mixed berries, banana, ground flaxseeds, Greek yogurt, and almond milk in a blender.
2. 2. Blend until smooth and creamy.
3. 3. Sweeten with honey or maple syrup if desired.
4. 4. Pour into a glass and serve immediately.

DESCRIPTION

This refreshing smoothie is packed with antioxidants from berries and omega-3 fatty acids from flaxseeds to support brain health and cognitive function.

Green Tea Matcha Latte

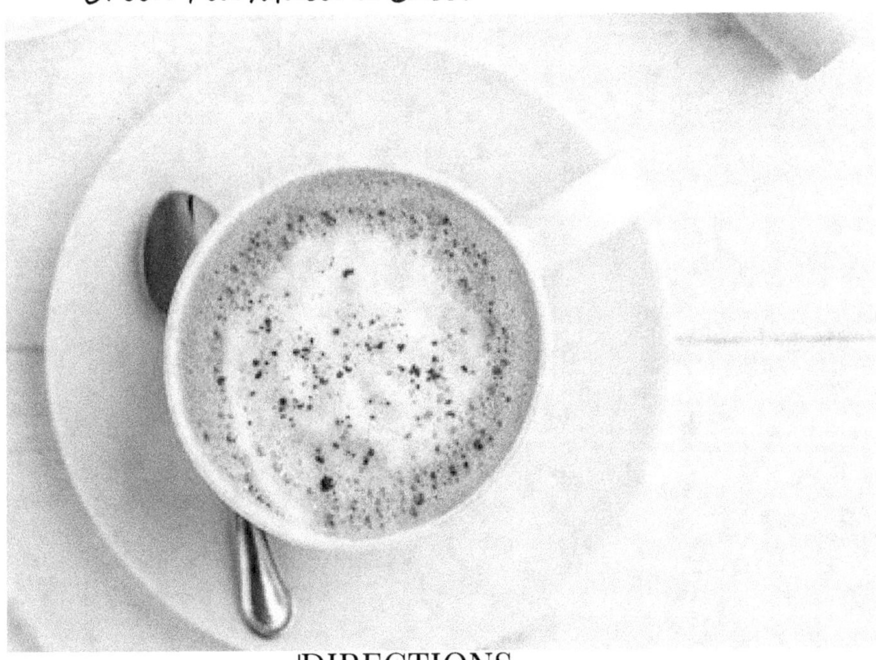

🍴 1 serving   🕐 5 minutes

INGREDIENTS

1 teaspoon matcha green
tea powder
1 cup almond milk
Honey or agave syrup to
taste (optional)

NUTRITIONAL VALUE

50 calories,
2g protein,
3g fat,
5g carbohydrates,
1g fiber.

DIRECTIONS

1. 1. In a small saucepan, heat almond milk over medium heat until warm but not boiling.
2. 2. Whisk in matcha green tea powder until dissolved and frothy.
3. 3. Sweeten with honey or agave syrup if desired.
4. 4. Pour into a mug and enjoy immediately.

DESCRIPTION

This creamy latte features antioxidant-rich matcha green tea powder and almond milk for a soothing and energizing beverage.

Citrus Infused Detox Water

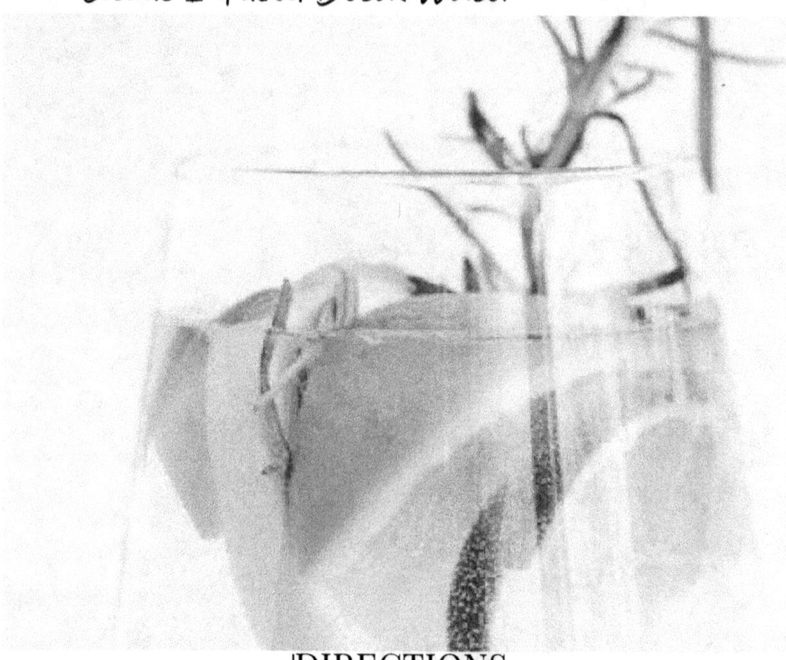

1 serving · **5 minutes**

INGREDIENTS

1/2 lemon, sliced

1/2 lime, sliced

1/2 orange, sliced

Few sprigs of fresh mint

2 cups water

NUTRITIONAL VALUE

0 calories,

0g protein,

0g fat,

0g carbohydrates,

0g fiber.

DIRECTIONS

1. 1. In a pitcher, combine lemon slices, lime slices, orange slices, and fresh mint.
2. 2. Add water and stir gently to combine.
3. 3. Refrigerate for at least 1 hour to allow the flavors to infuse.
4. 4. Serve over ice and enjoy.

DESCRIPTION

This infused water features citrus fruits and mint for a refreshing and hydrating beverage that helps detoxify the body and support overall health.

Turmeric Golden Milk

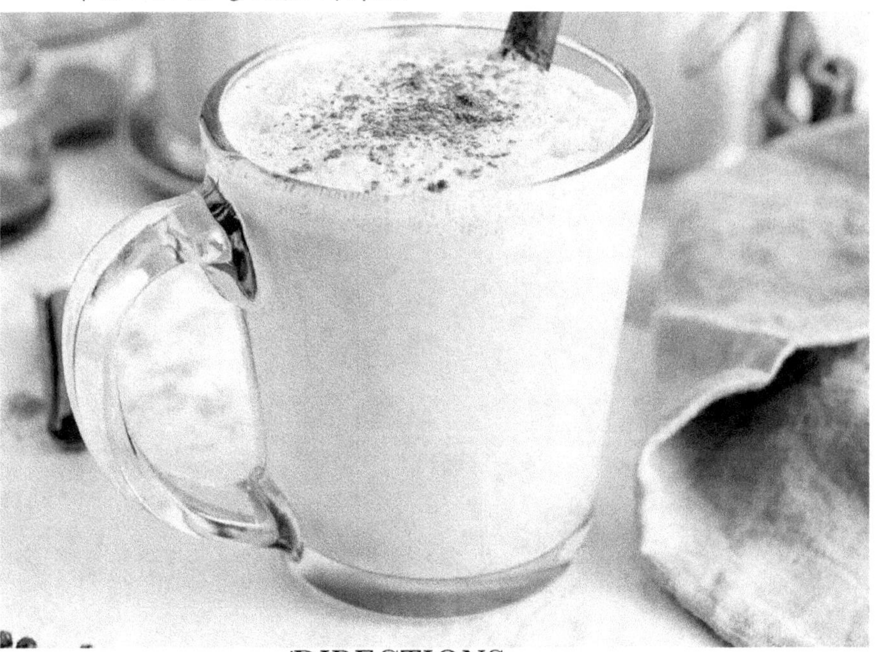

🍴 1 serving 🕐 10 minutes

INGREDIENTS

1 cup almond milk

1/2 teaspoon ground turmeric

1/4 teaspoon ground ginger

1/4 teaspoon ground cinnamon

Pinch of black pepper

Honey or maple syrup to taste

(optional)

NUTRITIONAL VALUE

50 calories,

1g protein,

3g fat,

5g carbohydrates,

1g fiber.

DIRECTIONS

1. 1. In a small saucepan, heat almond milk over medium heat until warm but not boiling.
2. 2. Whisk in ground turmeric, ground ginger, ground cinnamon, and black pepper until well combined.
3. 3. Sweeten with honey or maple syrup if desired.
4. 4. Pour into a mug and serve immediately.

DESCRIPTION

This warming beverage features turmeric, ginger, and cinnamon for their anti-inflammatory properties, promoting brain health and reducing oxidative stress.

Blueberry Brain Booster Smoothie

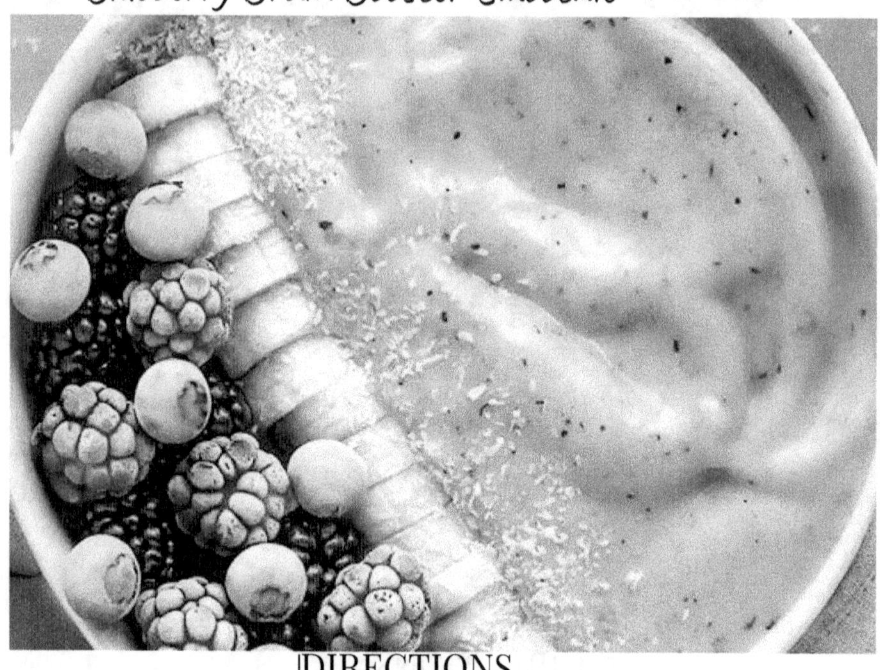

1 serving — 5 minutes

INGREDIENTS

2 cup frozen blueberries

1/2 banana

1/4 cup Greek yogurt

1/2 cup almond milk

1 tablespoon almond butter

1 teaspoon honey or maple syrup

(optional)

NUTRITIONAL VALUE

200 calories,

8g protein,

6g fat,

30g carbohydrates,

5g fiber.

DIRECTIONS

1. 1. Combine frozen blueberries, banana, Greek yogurt, almond milk, almond butter, and honey or maple syrup in a blender.

2. 2. Blend until smooth and creamy.

3. 3. Pour into a glass and serve immediately.

DESCRIPTION

This smoothie is loaded with blueberries, known for their high levels of antioxidants and their potential to improve memory and cognitive function.

Chamomile Lavender Tea

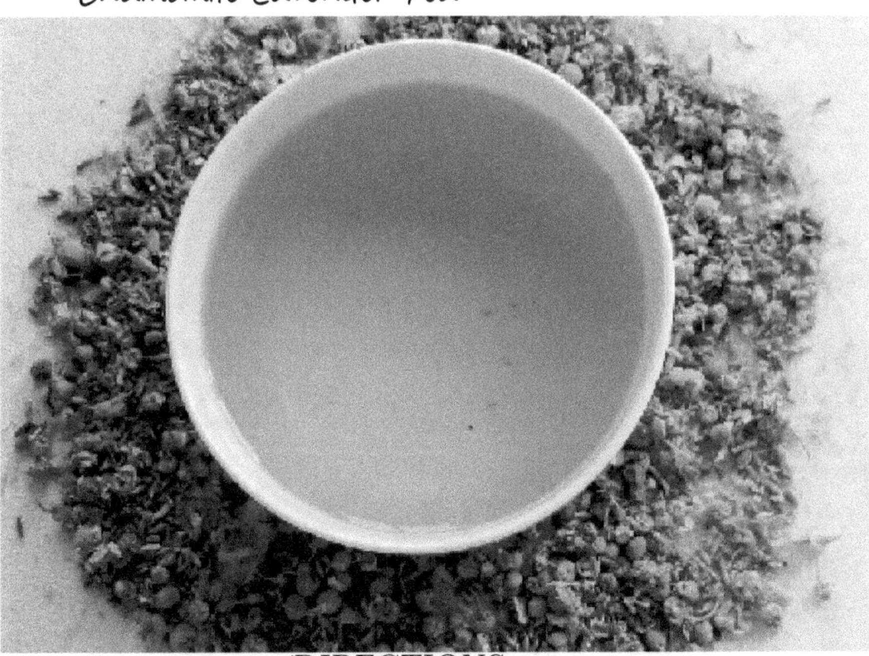

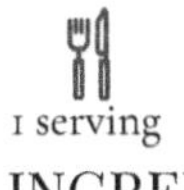

1 serving   5 minutes

INGREDIENTS

chamomile tea bag
1 teaspoon dried lavender
flowers
1 cup hot water
Honey or lemon to taste
(optional)

NUTRITIONAL VALUE

0 calories,
0g protein,
0g fat,
0g carbohydrates,
0g fiber.

DIRECTIONS

1. 1. Place chamomile tea bag and dried lavender flowers in a mug.

2. 2. Pour hot water over the tea bag and lavender flowers.

3. 3. Steep for 5 minutes, then remove the tea bag and lavender flowers.

4. 4. Sweeten with honey or add a squeeze of lemon if desired.

5. 5. Stir well and enjoy.

DESCRIPTION

This soothing herbal tea blend features chamomile and lavender, known for their calming properties, perfect for promoting relaxation and reducing stress.

Pineapple Ginger Immunity Juice

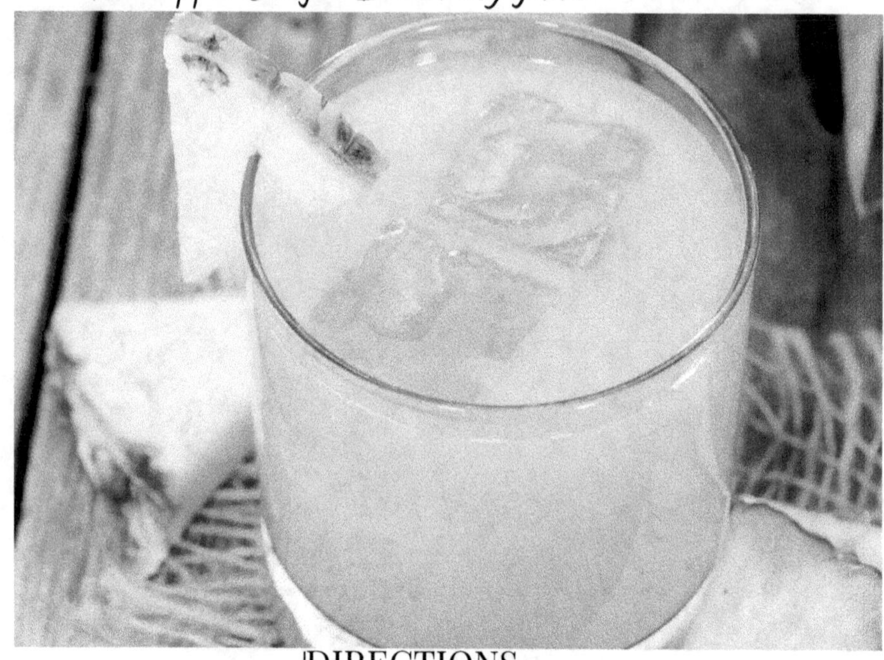

INGREDIENTS

1 serving   5 minutes

1 cup chopped pineapple

1-inch piece of ginger, peeled

1/2 lemon, peeled

1/2 cup water or coconut water

Ice cubes (optional)

NUTRITIONAL VALUE

200 calories,

5g protein,

15g fat,

15g carbohydrates,

3g fiber.

DIRECTIONS

1.1. Place chopped pineapple, peeled ginger, and peeled lemon in a blender.

2.2. Add water or coconut water.

3.3. Blend until smooth.

4.4. Strain the juice if desired.

5.5. Serve over ice cubes if desired.

6.6. Enjoy immediately.

DESCRIPTION

This invigorating juice blend features pineapple and ginger, known for their immune-boosting properties and anti-inflammatory benefits.

Coconut Water Berry Blast

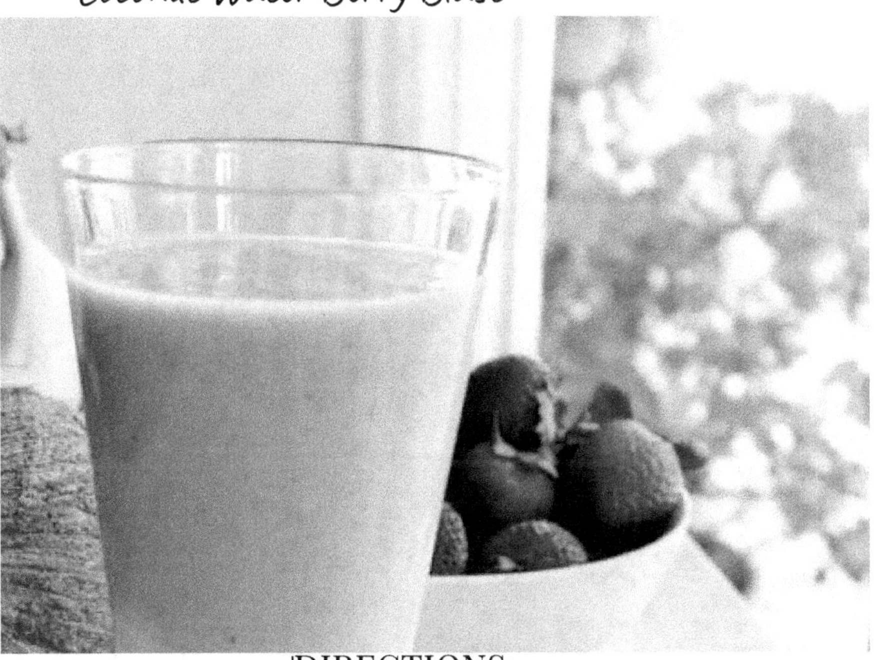

🍴 1 serving   🕐 5 minutes

INGREDIENTS

2 cup coconut water

1/2 cup mixed berries
(such as strawberries,
blueberries, and
raspberries)

Ice cubes (optional)

NUTRITIONAL VALUE

50 calories,
1g protein,
0g fat,
10g carbohydrates,
3g fiber.

DIRECTIONS

1. 1. In a blender, combine coconut water and mixed berries.
2. 2. Blend until smooth.
3. 3. Strain the mixture if desired.
4. 4. Serve over ice cubes if desired.
5. 5. Enjoy immediately.

DESCRIPTION

This hydrating beverage features coconut water and mixed berries for a refreshing and antioxidant-rich drink perfect for post-workout hydration.

Matcha Mint Iced Tea

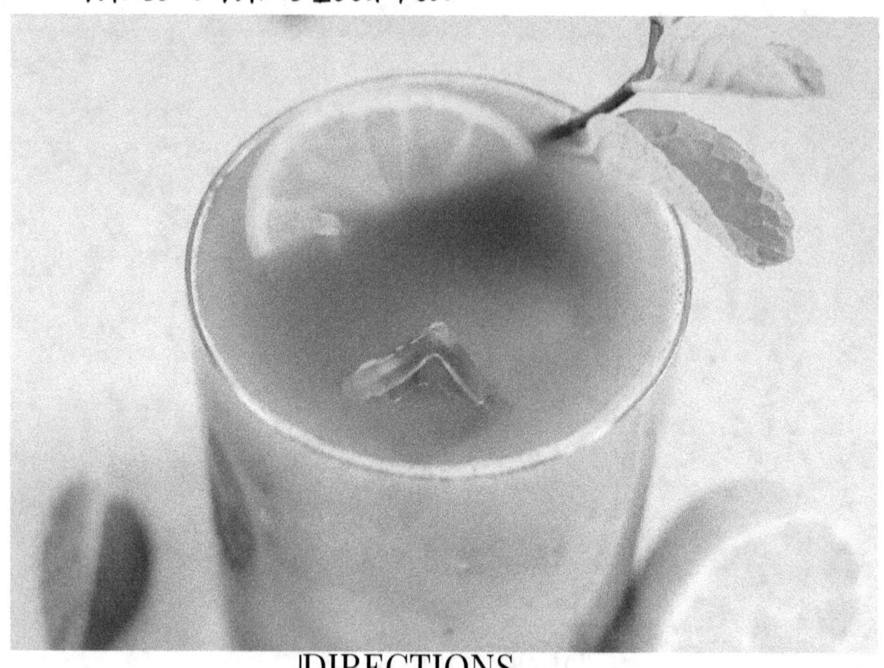

🍴 1 serving 🕐 5 minutes

INGREDIENTS

1 teaspoon matcha green tea powder

1 cup cold water

Fresh mint leaves

Honey or agave syrup to taste (optional)

Ice cubes

NUTRITIONAL VALUE

0 calories,

0g protein,

0g fat,

0g carbohydrates,

0g fiber.

DIRECTIONS

1. 1. In a glass, whisk matcha green tea powder with cold water until smooth.
2. 2. Add fresh mint leaves and sweeten with honey or agave syrup if desired.
3. 3. Stir well to combine.
4. 4. Add ice cubes to the glass.
5. 5. Serve immediately and enjoy.

DESCRIPTION

This refreshing iced tea features antioxidant-rich matcha green tea powder and fresh mint for a cooling and invigorating beverage.

Cocoa Almond Hot Chocolate

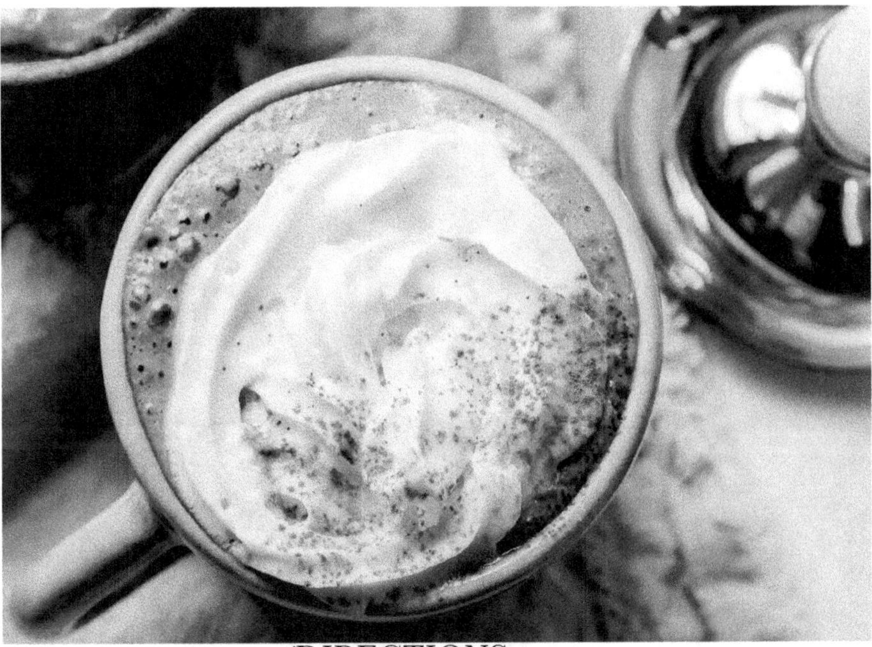

1 serving   5 minutes

INGREDIENTS

1 cup almond milk

2 tablespoons unsweetened cocoa powder

1 tablespoon honey or maple syrup

1/4 teaspoon vanilla extract

Pinch of salt

NUTRITIONAL VALUE

100 calories,

2g protein,

3g fat,

15g carbohydrates,

3g fiber.

DIRECTIONS

1.1. In a small saucepan, heat almond milk over medium heat until warm but not boiling.

2.2. Whisk in unsweetened cocoa powder, honey or maple syrup, vanilla extract, and a pinch of salt until smooth.

3.3. Continue to heat until hot, but not boiling.

4.4. Pour into a mug and serve immediately.

DESCRIPTION

This rich and creamy hot chocolate features cocoa powder and almond milk for a comforting and indulgent treat perfect for chilly days.

Special Occasions and Entertaining

Elegant Appetizers for Gatherings

Impressive Main Courses for Hosting

Delicious Sides to Accompany Any Meal

Indulgent Desserts for Celebrations

Caprese Skewers with Balsamic Glaze

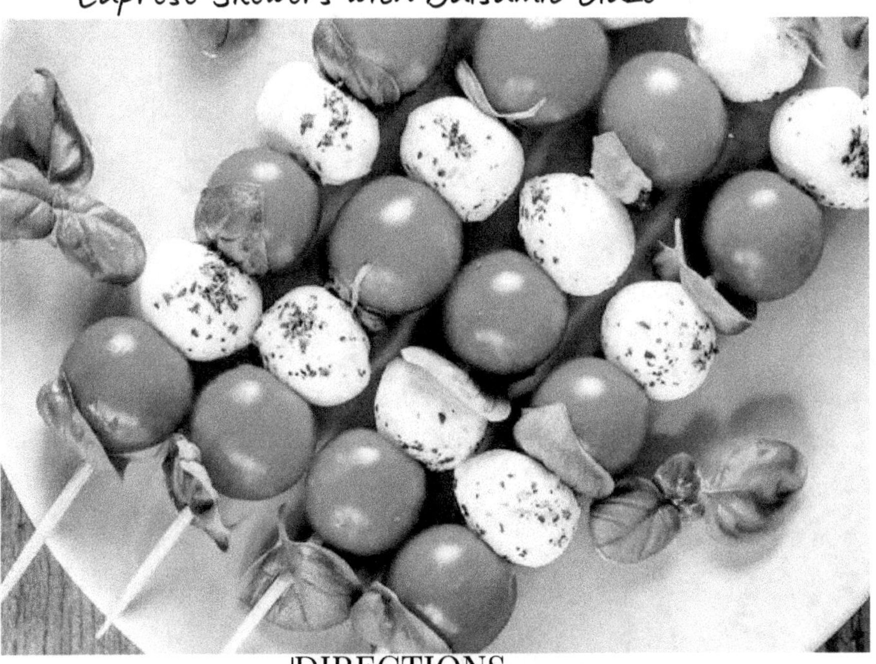

INGREDIENTS

Cherry tomatoes
Fresh mozzarella
balls
Fresh basil leaves
Balsamic glaze

NUTRITIONAL VALUE

50 calories,
2g protein,
4g fat,
2g carbohydrates,
1g fiber.

DIRECTIONS

1.1. Thread one cherry tomato, one fresh mozzarella ball, and one basil leaf onto each toothpick.

2.2. Arrange the skewers on a serving platter.

3.3. Drizzle with balsamic glaze just before serving.

4.4. Enjoy immediately.

DESCRIPTION

These elegant appetizers feature cherry tomatoes, fresh mozzarella balls, and basil leaves skewered on toothpicks and drizzled with a balsamic glaze.

Herb-Crusted Beef Tenderloin

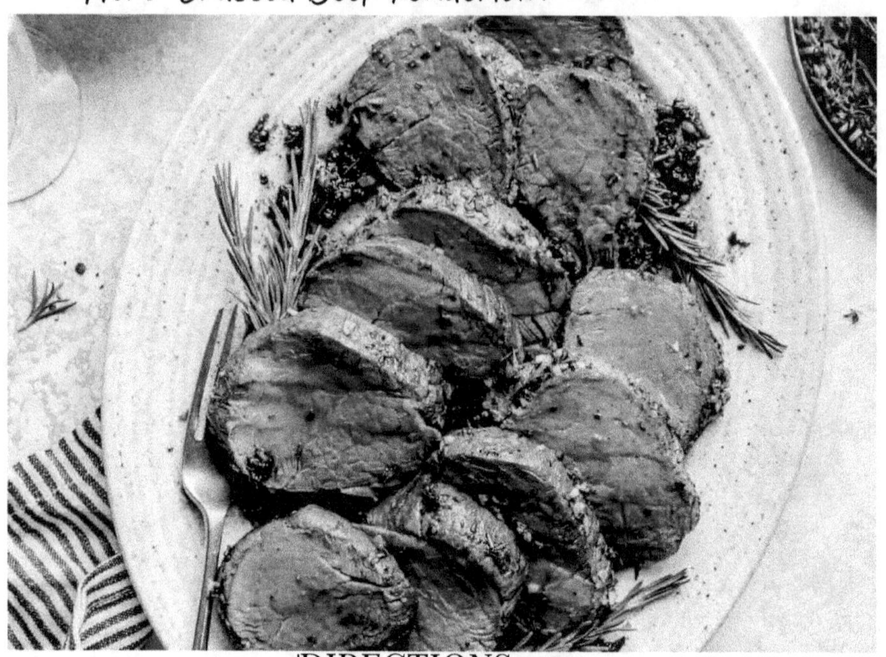

🍴 1 serving   🕐 30 minutes

INGREDIENTS

Beef tenderloin

Fresh herbs (such as rosemary, thyme, and parsley)

Garlic

Olive oil

Salt and pepper

NUTRITIONAL VALUE

300 calories,

25g protein,

20g fat,

0g carbohydrates,

0g fiber.

DIRECTIONS

1. 1. Preheat the oven to 425°F (220°C).
2. 2. In a food processor, combine fresh herbs, garlic, olive oil, salt, and pepper. Blend until a paste forms.
3. 3. Rub the herb mixture all over the beef tenderloin.
4. 4. Place the beef tenderloin on a roasting rack set in a roasting pan.
5. 5. Roast in the preheated oven for 25–30 minutes, or until the internal temperature reaches your desired doneness.
6. 6. Remove from the oven and let rest for 10 minutes before slicing.
7. 7. Serve sliced beef tenderloin with your favorite sides.

DESCRIPTION

This impressive main course features beef tenderloin coated in a flavorful herb crust and roasted to perfection.

Garlic Parmesan Roasted Potatoes

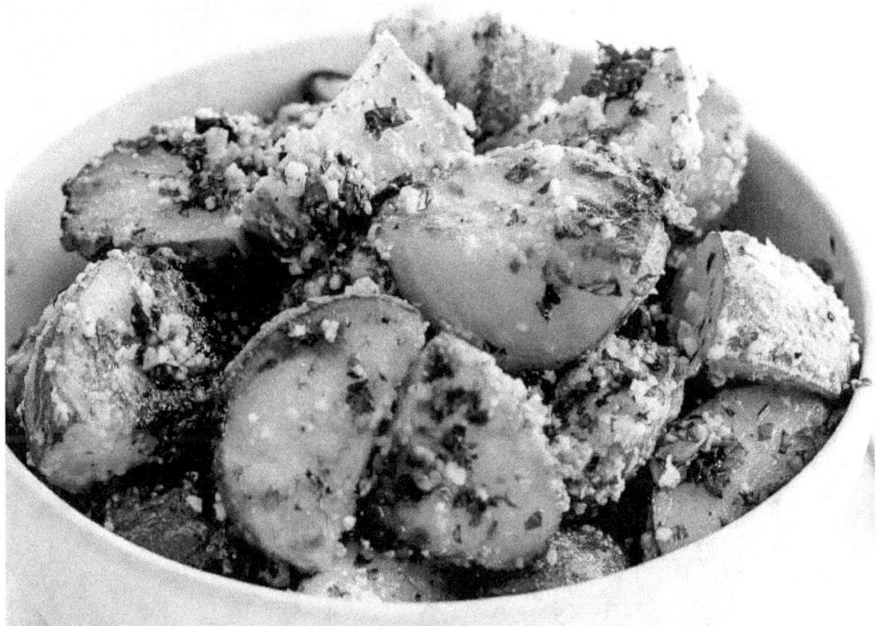

🍴 1 serving   🕐 30 minutes

INGREDIENTS

Potatoes

Garlic

Olive oil

Parmesan cheese

Fresh herbs (such as rosemary and thyme)

Salt and pepper

NUTRITIONAL VALUE

200 calories,

5g protein,

8g fat,

30g carbohydrates,

3g fiber.

DIRECTIONS

1.1. Preheat the oven to 425°F (220°C).

2.2. Cut potatoes into wedges or cubes and place them on a baking sheet.

3.3. Drizzle with olive oil and sprinkle with minced garlic, grated Parmesan cheese, chopped fresh herbs, salt, and pepper.

4.4. Toss to coat evenly.

5.5. Roast in the preheated oven for 25-30 minutes, or until golden and crispy.

6.6. Serve hot and enjoy.

DESCRIPTION

These delicious roasted potatoes are tossed with garlic, Parmesan cheese, and fresh herbs for a flavorful side dish that pairs well with any meal.

Chocolate Lava Cakes

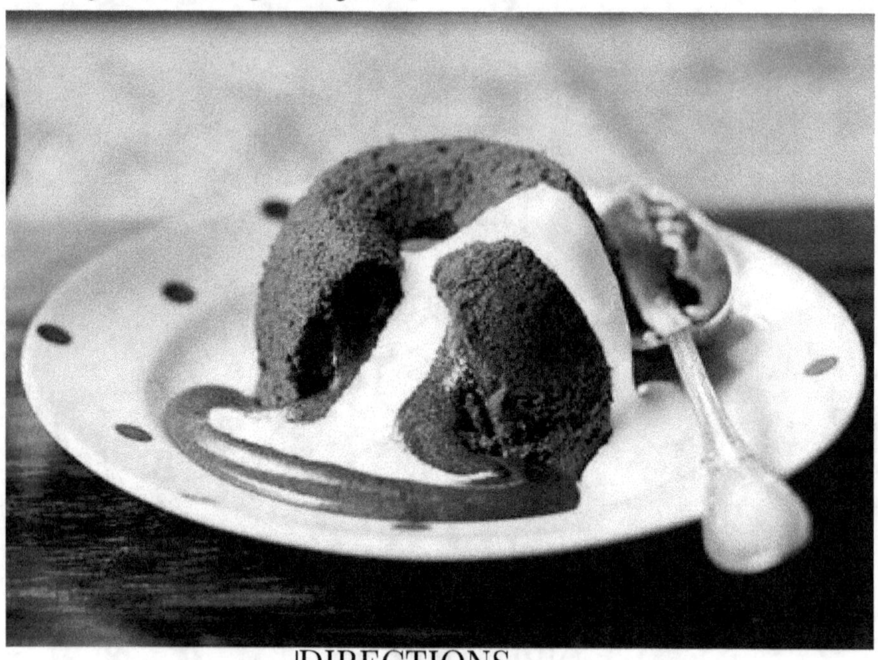

1 cake   12 minutes

INGREDIENTS

Dark chocolate

Butter

Eggs

Sugar

Flour

Salt

Vanilla extract

NUTRITIONAL VALUE

300 calories,

5g protein,

20g fat,

30g carbohydrates,

3g fiber.

DIRECTIONS

1.1. Preheat the oven to 425°F (220°C). Grease and flour individual ramekins.

2.2. In a microwave-safe bowl, melt dark chocolate and butter together. Stir until smooth.

3.3. In a separate bowl, whisk together eggs, sugar, flour, salt, and vanilla extract until well combined.

4.4. Stir the melted chocolate mixture into the egg mixture until smooth.

5.5. Divide the batter evenly among the prepared ramekins.

6.6. Place the ramekins on a baking sheet and bake in the preheated oven for 12 minutes.

7.7. Remove from the oven and let cool for 1 minute.

8.8. Carefully invert the cakes onto serving plates.

9.9. Serve immediately, garnished with powdered sugar or a scoop of vanilla ice cream if desired.

DESCRIPTION

These indulgent desserts feature rich chocolate cake with a gooey molten center, perfect for celebrating special occasions.

Prosciutto-Wrapped Asparagus

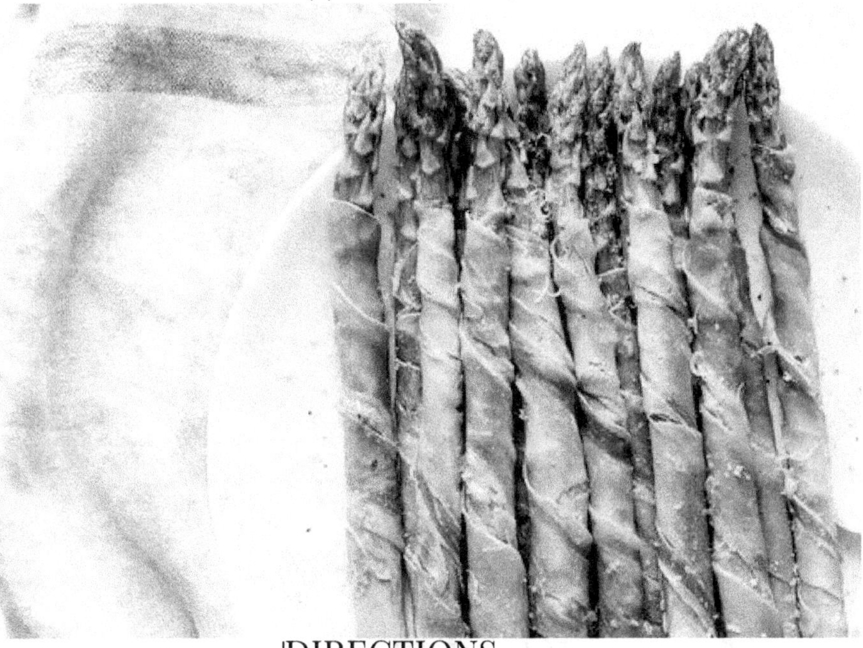

1 serving   **10 minutes**

INGREDIENTS

Asparagus spears

Prosciutto slices

Olive oil

Salt and pepper

NUTRITIONAL VALUE
100 calories,
2g protein,
3g fat,
15g carbohydrates,
3g fiber.

DIRECTIONS

1.1. Preheat the oven to 400°F (200°C).
2.2. Trim the woody ends off the asparagus spears.
3.3. Wrap each asparagus spear with a slice of prosciutto.
4.4. Place the wrapped asparagus spears on a baking sheet.
5.5. Drizzle with olive oil and season with salt and pepper.
6.6. Roast in the preheated oven for 8-10 minutes, or until the asparagus is tender and the prosciutto is crispy.
7.7. Serve hot and enjoy.

DESCRIPTION

These elegant appetizers feature tender asparagus spears wrapped in salty prosciutto, perfect for entertaining guests.

Herb-Crusted Salmon Fillets

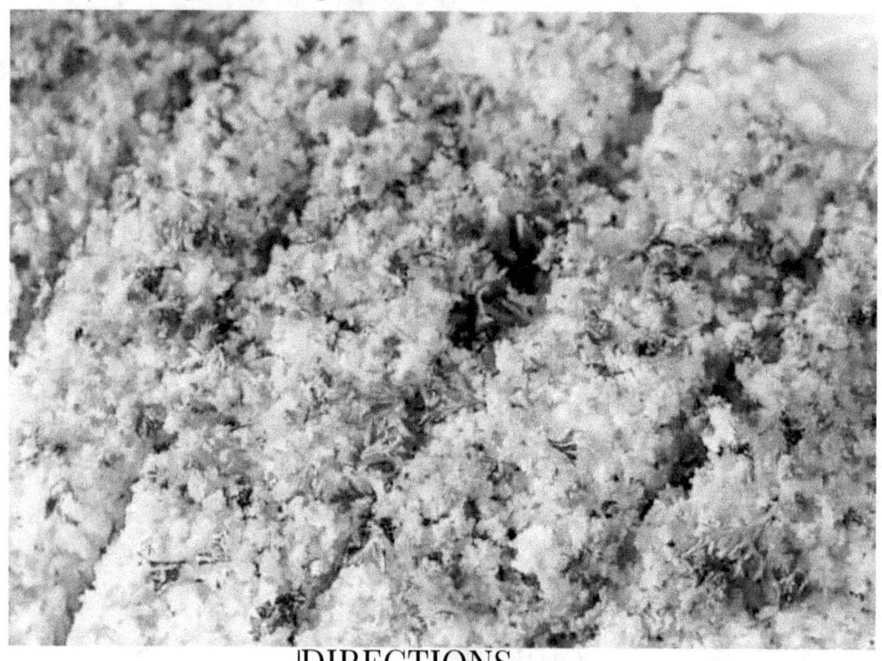

1 serving **15 minutes**

INGREDIENTS

Salmon fillets

Fresh herbs (such as dill, parsley, and chives)

Garlic

Olive oil

Lemon

Salt and pepper

NUTRITIONAL VALUE

250 calories,

25g protein,

15g fat,

0g carbohydrates,

0g fiber.

DIRECTIONS

1. 1. Preheat the oven to 400°F (200°C).
2. 2. In a food processor, combine fresh herbs, garlic, olive oil, lemon zest, salt, and pepper. Blend until a paste forms.
3. 3. Rub the herb mixture all over the salmon fillets.
4. 4. Place the salmon fillets on a baking sheet lined with parchment paper.
5. 5. Bake in the preheated oven for 12–15 minutes, or until the salmon is cooked through and flakes easily with a fork.
6. 6. Serve hot with lemon wedges.

DESCRIPTION

These impressive main courses feature salmon fillets coated in a flavorful herb crust and baked to perfection.

Roasted Brussels Sprouts with Bacon

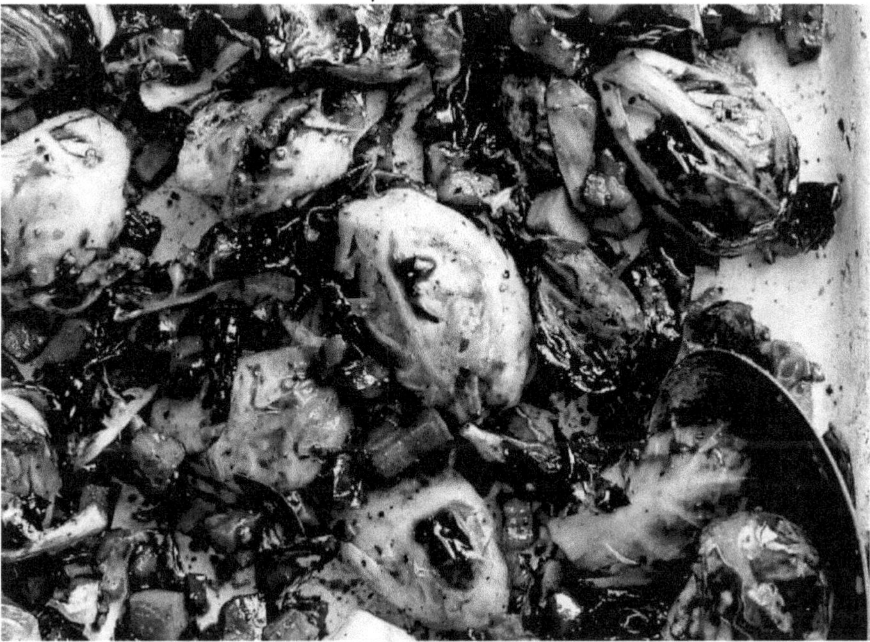

INGREDIENTS

Brussels sprouts
Bacon strips
Olive oil
Balsamic vinegar
Salt and pepper

NUTRITIONAL VALUE

150 calories,
5g protein,
10g fat,
10g carbohydrates,
5g fiber.

DIRECTIONS

1. 1. Preheat the oven to 400°F (200°C).
2. 2. Trim the ends off the Brussels sprouts and cut them in half.
3. 3. Place the Brussels sprouts on a baking sheet lined with parchment paper.
4. 4. Drizzle with olive oil and toss to coat evenly.
5. 5. Season with salt and pepper.
6. 6. Arrange the bacon strips on top of the Brussels sprouts.
7. 7. Roast in the preheated oven for 20-25 minutes, or until the Brussels sprouts are golden and crispy.
8. 8. Drizzle with balsamic vinegar before serving.

DESCRIPTION

These delicious sides feature Brussels sprouts roasted to perfection with crispy bacon for added flavor and texture.

Decadent Flourless Chocolate Cake

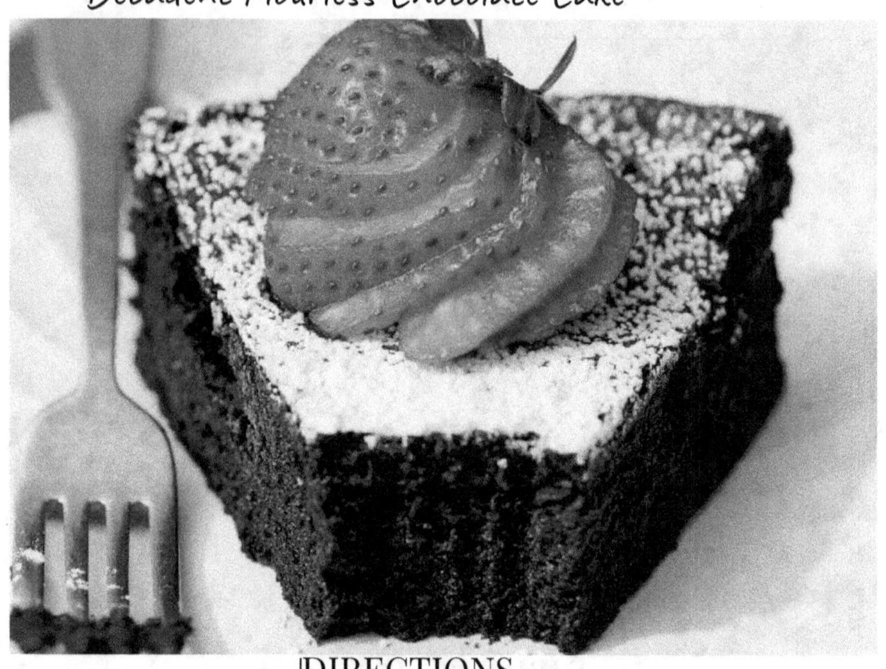

🍴 1 slice   🕐 30 minutes

INGREDIENTS

Dark chocolate

Butter

Eggs

Sugar

Cocoa powder

Vanilla extract

Salt

NUTRITIONAL VALUE

300 calories,

5g protein,

20g fat,

25g carbohydrates,

3g fiber.

DIRECTIONS

1.1. Preheat the oven to 350°F (180°C). Grease and flour a round cake pan.

2.2. In a heatproof bowl set over a pot of simmering water, melt dark chocolate and butter together. Stir until smooth.

3.3. In a separate bowl, whisk together eggs, sugar, cocoa powder, vanilla extract, and salt until well combined.

4.4. Stir the melted chocolate mixture into the egg mixture until smooth.

5.5. Pour the batter into the prepared cake pan.

6.6. Bake in the preheated oven for 25-30 minutes, or until the edges are set but the center is still slightly jiggly.

7.7. Remove from the oven and let cool in the pan for 10 minutes.

8.8. Carefully invert the cake onto a serving plate.

9.9. Serve warm or at room temperature, garnished with powdered sugar or whipped cream if desired.

DESCRIPTION

This indulgent dessert features rich and fudgy chocolate cake made without flour, perfect for satisfying your sweet tooth.

Stuffed Mushrooms with Cream Cheese and Spinach

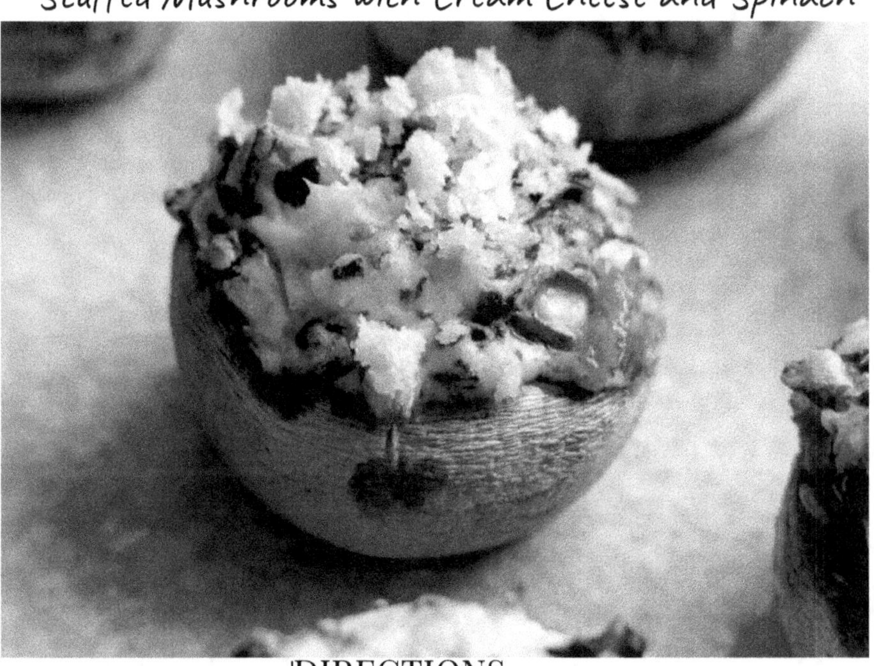

1 serving   20 minutes

INGREDIENTS

Mushrooms

Cream cheese

Spinach

Garlic

Parmesan cheese

Bread crumbs

Olive oil

Salt and pepper

NUTRITIONAL VALUE

100 calories,

3g protein,

8g fat,

5g carbohydrates,

2g fiber.

DIRECTIONS

1.1. Preheat the oven to 375°F (190°C). Grease a baking dish with olive oil.

2.2. Remove the stems from the mushrooms and set aside.

3.3. In a skillet, sauté the mushroom stems, spinach, and minced garlic until the spinach is wilted.

4.4. In a bowl, combine cream cheese, sautéed spinach mixture, grated Parmesan cheese, bread crumbs, salt, and pepper.

5.5. Stuff each mushroom cap with the cream cheese mixture.

6.6. Place the stuffed mushrooms in the prepared baking dish.

7.7. Bake in the preheated oven for 15-20 minutes, or until the mushrooms are tender and the filling is golden and bubbly.

8.8. Serve hot and enjoy.

DESCRIPTION

These elegant appetizers feature mushrooms stuffed with a creamy mixture of cream cheese, spinach, and garlic.

Classic Tiramisu

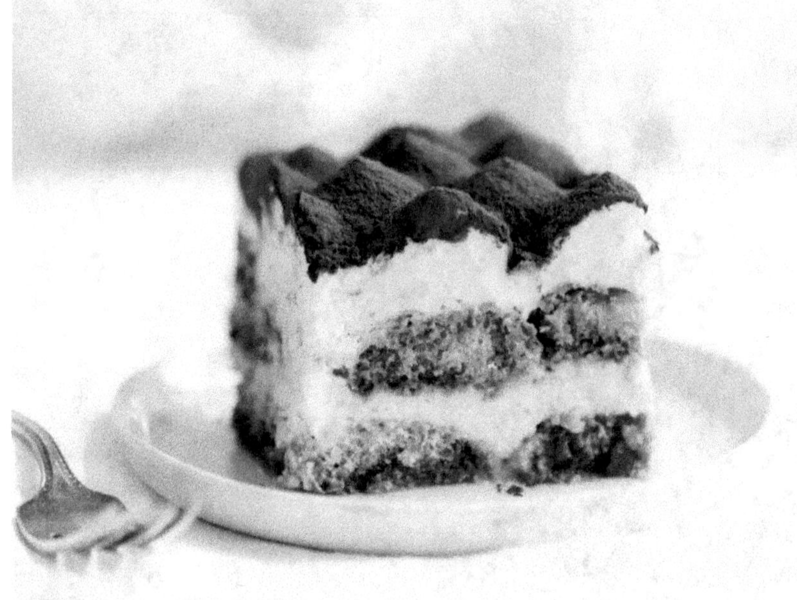

1 slice   30 minutes

INGREDIENTS

Ladyfingers

Espresso coffee

Mascarpone cheese

Eggs

Sugar

Marsala wine or rum

Cocoa powder

NUTRITIONAL VALUE

250 calories,

5g protein,

15g fat,

20g carbohydrates,

1g fiber.

DIRECTIONS

1.1. Brew espresso coffee and let it cool to room temperature.

2.2. In a bowl, whisk together mascarpone cheese, egg yolks, sugar, and Marsala wine or rum until smooth.

3.3. In a separate bowl, beat egg whites until stiff peaks form.

4.4. Gently fold the beaten egg whites into the mascarpone mixture until well combined.

5.5. Dip each ladyfinger into the cooled espresso coffee and arrange them in a single layer in the bottom of a serving dish.

6.6. Spread half of the mascarpone mixture over the ladyfingers.

7.7. Repeat with another layer of dipped ladyfingers and the remaining mascarpone mixture.

8.8. Cover and refrigerate for at least 4 hours or overnight to set.

9.9. Before serving, dust the top of the tiramisu with cocoa powder.

10.10. Serve chilled and enjoy.

DESCRIPTION

This classic Italian dessert features layers of coffee-soaked ladyfingers and mascarpone cheese filling, dusted with cocoa powder for a decadent treat.

Conclusion

In our journey toward enhancing brain health and promoting cognitive wellness, we've explored various strategies and practices that can make a significant difference in maintaining mental acuity and overall well-being. Here's a recap of the key points discussed:

1. Nutrition for Brain Health: We've learned about the importance of incorporating nutrient-rich foods into our diet, such as omega-3 fatty acids, antioxidants, vitamins, and minerals, which play crucial roles in supporting cognitive function and brain health.

2. Lifestyle Factors: We've examined the impact of lifestyle factors, including regular exercise, stress management techniques, nurturing social connections, and engaging in stimulating mental activities and hobbies, on brain health and cognitive wellness.

3. Practical Tips: We've provided practical tips for stocking a brain-boosting pantry, meal planning, and preparation, as well as suggestions for kitchen tools and gadgets that can aid in preparing brain-healthy recipes.

4. Delicious Recipes: We've curated a collection of delicious and nutritious recipes for breakfasts, lunches, dinners, snacks, beverages, and special occasions, designed to support brain health and delight the taste buds.

5. Committing to a Brain-Healthy Lifestyle: Finally, we've emphasized the importance of committing to a brain-healthy lifestyle by incorporating these strategies and practices into our daily routines. By making conscious choices to prioritize brain health, we can enhance cognitive function, reduce the risk of age-related cognitive decline, and enjoy a higher quality of life.

The meal plans provided can work effectively for a week, offering two days' worth of breakfast, lunch, dinner, and snacks. You can rotate between the provided meal options for each day of the week, allowing for variety while still adhering to your dietary preferences and goals. If you prefer more variety or want to extend the meal plan for a longer duration, you can mix and match the recipes or repeat the meal plan for subsequent weeks. Additionally, you can use the meal plan as a template and make adjustments based on seasonal ingredients, personal taste preferences, or specific nutritional needs. Ultimately, the duration of the meal plan depends on individual preferences and dietary requirements.

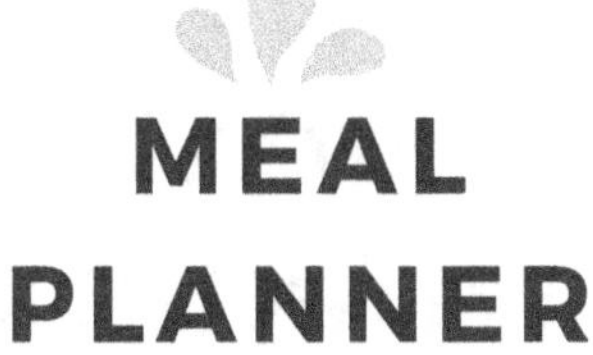

MEAL
PLANNER

DAY 1

- Breakfast: Energizing Smoothie Bowl
- Lunch: Colorful Grain Salad
- Dinner: Plant-Powered Main Course - Herb-Crusted Salmon Fillets
- Snack: Energy-Boosting Nut and Seed Mix

DAY 2

- Breakfast: Nutrient-Packed Oatmeal Variation
- Lunch: Wholesome Wrap and Sandwich Creation - Stuffed Mushrooms with Cream Cheese and Spinach
- Dinner: Comforting Grain and Pasta Recipe - Garlic Parmesan Roasted Potatoes
- Snack: Guilt-Free Dip and Spread Recipe - Hummus with Veggie Sticks

Vegan Meal Plan

DAY 1

- Breakfast: Energizing Smoothie Bowl
- Lunch: Vibrant Buddha Bowl
- Dinner: Plant-Powered Main Course - Herb-Crusted Salmon Fillets (substitute with tofu or tempeh)
- Snack: Energy-Boosting Nut and Seed Mix

DAY 2

- Breakfast: Nutrient-Packed Oatmeal Variation
- Lunch: Colorful Grain Salad
- Dinner: Comforting Grain and Pasta Recipe - Garlic Parmesan Roasted Potatoes (use vegan cheese)
- Snack: Guilt-Free Dip and Spread Recipe - Baba Ganoush with Veggie Sticks

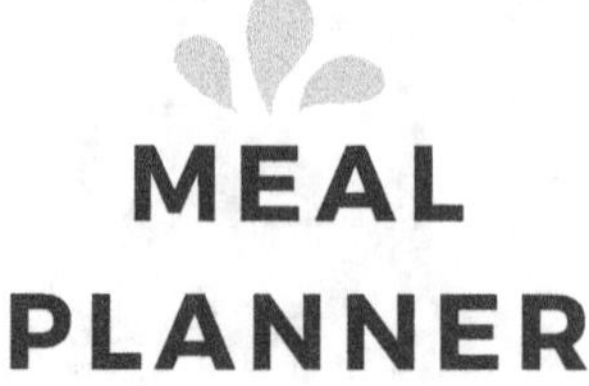

MEAL PLANNER

VEGETARIAN MEAL PLAN

DAY 1

- Breakfast: Energizing Smoothie Bowl
- Lunch: Colorful Grain Salad
- Dinner: Plant-Powered Main Course - Herb-Crusted Salmon Fillets
- Snack: Energy-Boosting Nut and Seed Mix

DAY 2

- Breakfast: Nutrient-Packed Oatmeal Variation
- Lunch: Wholesome Wrap and Sandwich Creation - Stuffed Mushrooms with Cream Cheese and Spinach
- Dinner: Comforting Grain and Pasta Recipe - Garlic Parmesan Roasted Potatoes
- Snack: Guilt-Free Dip and Spread Recipe - Hummus with Veggie Sticks

Vegan Meal Plan

DAY 1

- Breakfast: Energizing Smoothie Bowl
- Lunch: Vibrant Buddha Bowl
- Dinner: Plant-Powered Main Course - Herb-Crusted Salmon Fillets (substitute with tofu or tempeh)
- Snack: Energy-Boosting Nut and Seed Mix

DAY 2

- Breakfast: Nutrient-Packed Oatmeal Variation
- Lunch: Colorful Grain Salad
- Dinner: Comforting Grain and Pasta Recipe - Garlic Parmesan Roasted Potatoes (use vegan cheese)
- Snack: Guilt-Free Dip and Spread Recipe - Baba Ganoush with Veggie Sticks

MEAL PLANNER

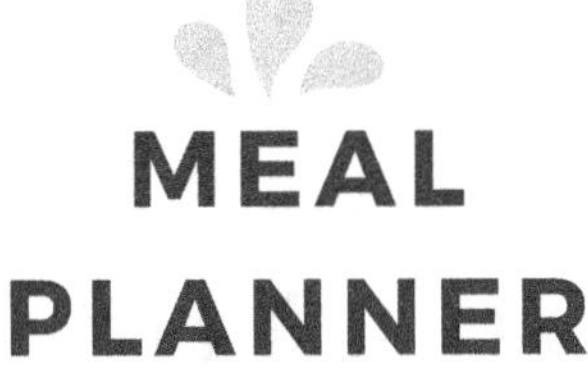

VEGETARIAN MEAL PLAN

DAY 1

- Breakfast: Energizing Smoothie Bowl
- Lunch: Colorful Grain Salad
- Dinner: Plant-Powered Main Course - Herb-Crusted Salmon Fillets
- Snack: Energy-Boosting Nut and Seed Mix

DAY 2

- Breakfast: Nutrient-Packed Oatmeal Variation
- Lunch: Wholesome Wrap and Sandwich Creation - Stuffed Mushrooms with Cream Cheese and Spinach
- Dinner: Comforting Grain and Pasta Recipe - Garlic Parmesan Roasted Potatoes
- Snack: Guilt-Free Dip and Spread Recipe - Hummus with Veggie Sticks

Vegan Meal Plan

DAY 1

- Breakfast: Energizing Smoothie Bowl
- Lunch: Vibrant Buddha Bowl
- Dinner: Plant-Powered Main Course - Herb-Crusted Salmon Fillets (substitute with tofu or tempeh)
- Snack: Energy-Boosting Nut and Seed Mix

DAY 2

- Breakfast: Nutrient-Packed Oatmeal Variation
- Lunch: Colorful Grain Salad
- Dinner: Comforting Grain and Pasta Recipe - Garlic Parmesan Roasted Potatoes (use vegan cheese)
- Snack: Guilt-Free Dip and Spread Recipe - Baba Ganoush with Veggie Sticks

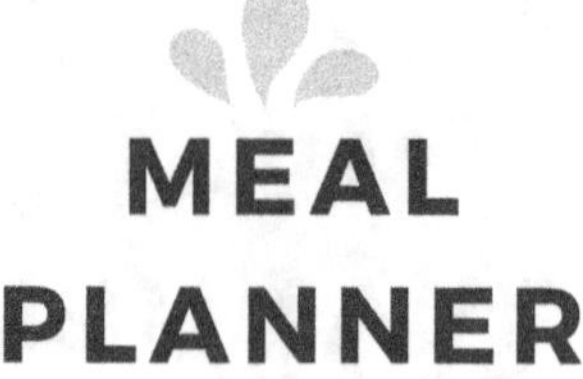

MEAL PLANNER

VEGETARIAN MEAL PLAN

DAY 1

- Breakfast: Energizing Smoothie Bowl
- Lunch: Colorful Grain Salad
- Dinner: Plant-Powered Main Course - Herb-Crusted Salmon Fillets
- Snack: Energy-Boosting Nut and Seed Mix

DAY 2

- Breakfast: Nutrient-Packed Oatmeal Variation
- Lunch: Wholesome Wrap and Sandwich Creation - Stuffed Mushrooms with Cream Cheese and Spinach
- Dinner: Comforting Grain and Pasta Recipe - Garlic Parmesan Roasted Potatoes
- Snack: Guilt-Free Dip and Spread Recipe - Hummus with Veggie Sticks

Vegan Meal Plan

DAY 1

- Breakfast: Energizing Smoothie Bowl
- Lunch: Vibrant Buddha Bowl
- Dinner: Plant-Powered Main Course - Herb-Crusted Salmon Fillets (substitute with tofu or tempeh)
- Snack: Energy-Boosting Nut and Seed Mix

DAY 2

- Breakfast: Nutrient-Packed Oatmeal Variation
- Lunch: Colorful Grain Salad
- Dinner: Comforting Grain and Pasta Recipe - Garlic Parmesan Roasted Potatoes (use vegan cheese)
- Snack: Guilt-Free Dip and Spread Recipe - Baba Ganoush with Veggie Sticks

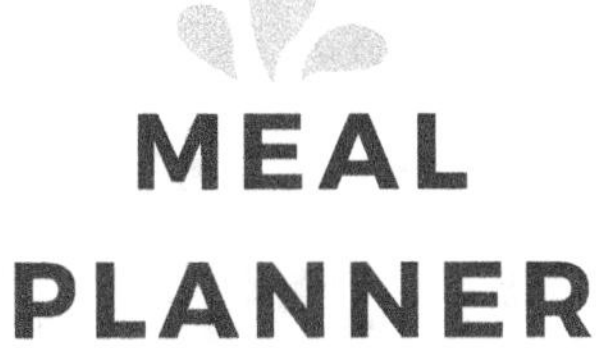

MEAL
PLANNER

DAY 1

- Breakfast: Energizing Smoothie Bowl
- Lunch: Colorful Grain Salad
- Dinner: Plant-Powered Main Course - Herb-Crusted Salmon Fillets
- Snack: Energy-Boosting Nut and Seed Mix

DAY 2

- Breakfast: Nutrient-Packed Oatmeal Variation
- Lunch: Wholesome Wrap and Sandwich Creation - Stuffed Mushrooms with Cream Cheese and Spinach
- Dinner: Comforting Grain and Pasta Recipe - Garlic Parmesan Roasted Potatoes
- Snack: Guilt-Free Dip and Spread Recipe - Hummus with Veggie Sticks

Vegan Meal Plan

DAY 1

- Breakfast: Energizing Smoothie Bowl
- Lunch: Vibrant Buddha Bowl
- Dinner: Plant-Powered Main Course - Herb-Crusted Salmon Fillets (substitute with tofu or tempeh)
- Snack: Energy-Boosting Nut and Seed Mix

DAY 2

- Breakfast: Nutrient-Packed Oatmeal Variation
- Lunch: Colorful Grain Salad
- Dinner: Comforting Grain and Pasta Recipe - Garlic Parmesan Roasted Potatoes (use vegan cheese)
- Snack: Guilt-Free Dip and Spread Recipe - Baba Ganoush with Veggie Sticks

MEAL PLANNER

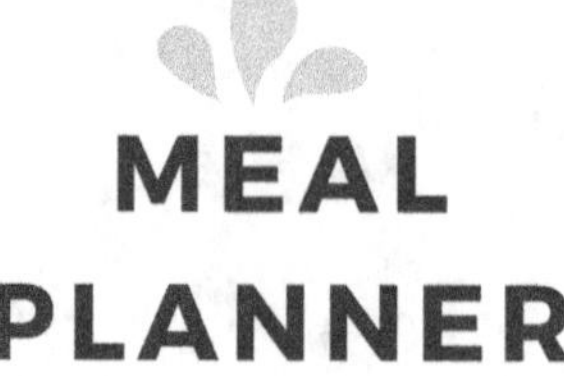

DAY 1

- Breakfast: Energizing Smoothie Bowl (ensure all ingredients are gluten-free)
- Lunch: Colorful Grain Salad (use gluten-free grains)
- Dinner: Flavorful Fish and Seafood Dish - Herb-Crusted Salmon Fillets
- Snack: Energy-Boosting Nut and Seed Mix

DAY 2

- Breakfast: Nutrient-Packed Oatmeal Variation (use gluten-free oats)
- Lunch: Wholesome Wrap and Sandwich Creation - Stuffed Mushrooms with Cream Cheese and Spinach (ensure all ingredients are gluten-free)
- Dinner: Comforting Grain and Pasta Recipe - Garlic Parmesan Roasted Potatoes (use gluten-free breadcrumbs)
- Snack: Guilt-Free Dip and Spread Recipe - Hummus with Veggie Sticks

Paleo Meal Plan

DAY 1

- Breakfast: Protein-Packed Breakfast Burritos (use lettuce wraps instead of tortillas)
- Lunch: Satisfying Soup and Stew Recipe - Roasted Brussels Sprouts with Bacon
- Dinner: Flavorful Fish and Seafood Dish - Herb-Crusted Salmon Fillets
- Snack: Energy-Boosting Nut and Seed Mix

DAY 2

- Breakfast: Nutrient-Packed Oatmeal Variation (use nuts and seeds instead of oats)
- Lunch: Wholesome Wrap and Sandwich Creation - Prosciutto-Wrapped Asparagus
- Dinner: Comforting Grain and Pasta Recipe - Zucchini Noodles with Pesto
- Snack: Guilt-Free Dip and Spread Recipe - Guacamole with Veggie Sticks

MEAL PLANNER

GLUTEN-FREE MEAL PLAN

DAY 1

- Breakfast: Energizing Smoothie Bowl (ensure all ingredients are gluten-free)
- Lunch: Colorful Grain Salad (use gluten-free grains)
- Dinner: Flavorful Fish and Seafood Dish - Herb-Crusted Salmon Fillets
- Snack: Energy-Boosting Nut and Seed Mix

DAY 2

- Breakfast: Nutrient-Packed Oatmeal Variation (use gluten-free oats)
- Lunch: Wholesome Wrap and Sandwich Creation - Stuffed Mushrooms with Cream Cheese and Spinach (ensure all ingredients are gluten-free)
- Dinner: Comforting Grain and Pasta Recipe - Garlic Parmesan Roasted Potatoes (use gluten-free breadcrumbs)
- Snack: Guilt-Free Dip and Spread Recipe - Hummus with Veggie Sticks

Paleo Meal Plan

DAY 1

- Breakfast: Protein-Packed Breakfast Burritos (use lettuce wraps instead of tortillas)
- Lunch: Satisfying Soup and Stew Recipe - Roasted Brussels Sprouts with Bacon
- Dinner: Flavorful Fish and Seafood Dish - Herb-Crusted Salmon Fillets
- Snack: Energy-Boosting Nut and Seed Mix

DAY 2

- Breakfast: Nutrient-Packed Oatmeal Variation (use nuts and seeds instead of oats)
- Lunch: Wholesome Wrap and Sandwich Creation - Prosciutto-Wrapped Asparagus
- Dinner: Comforting Grain and Pasta Recipe - Zucchini Noodles with Pesto
- Snack: Guilt-Free Dip and Spread Recipe - Guacamole with Veggie Sticks

MEAL PLANNER

GLUTEN-FREE MEAL PLAN

DAY 1

- Breakfast: Energizing Smoothie Bowl (ensure all ingredients are gluten-free)
- Lunch: Colorful Grain Salad (use gluten-free grains)
- Dinner: Flavorful Fish and Seafood Dish - Herb-Crusted Salmon Fillets
- Snack: Energy-Boosting Nut and Seed Mix

DAY 2

- Breakfast: Nutrient-Packed Oatmeal Variation (use gluten-free oats)
- Lunch: Wholesome Wrap and Sandwich Creation - Stuffed Mushrooms with Cream Cheese and Spinach (ensure all ingredients are gluten-free)
- Dinner: Comforting Grain and Pasta Recipe - Garlic Parmesan Roasted Potatoes (use gluten-free breadcrumbs)
- Snack: Guilt-Free Dip and Spread Recipe - Hummus with Veggie Sticks

Paleo Meal Plan

DAY 1

- Breakfast: Protein-Packed Breakfast Burritos (use lettuce wraps instead of tortillas)
- Lunch: Satisfying Soup and Stew Recipe - Roasted Brussels Sprouts with Bacon
- Dinner: Flavorful Fish and Seafood Dish - Herb-Crusted Salmon Fillets
- Snack: Energy-Boosting Nut and Seed Mix

DAY 2

- Breakfast: Nutrient-Packed Oatmeal Variation (use nuts and seeds instead of oats)
- Lunch: Wholesome Wrap and Sandwich Creation - Prosciutto-Wrapped Asparagus
- Dinner: Comforting Grain and Pasta Recipe - Zucchini Noodles with Pesto
- Snack: Guilt-Free Dip and Spread Recipe - Guacamole with Veggie Sticks

MEAL PLANNER

DAY 1

- Breakfast: Energizing Smoothie Bowl (ensure all ingredients are gluten-free)
- Lunch: Colorful Grain Salad (use gluten-free grains)
- Dinner: Flavorful Fish and Seafood Dish - Herb-Crusted Salmon Fillets
- Snack: Energy-Boosting Nut and Seed Mix

DAY 2

- Breakfast: Nutrient-Packed Oatmeal Variation (use gluten-free oats)
- Lunch: Wholesome Wrap and Sandwich Creation - Stuffed Mushrooms with Cream Cheese and Spinach (ensure all ingredients are gluten-free)
- Dinner: Comforting Grain and Pasta Recipe - Garlic Parmesan Roasted Potatoes (use gluten-free breadcrumbs)
- Snack: Guilt-Free Dip and Spread Recipe - Hummus with Veggie Sticks

Paleo Meal Plan

DAY 1

- Breakfast: Protein-Packed Breakfast Burritos (use lettuce wraps instead of tortillas)
- Lunch: Satisfying Soup and Stew Recipe - Roasted Brussels Sprouts with Bacon
- Dinner: Flavorful Fish and Seafood Dish - Herb-Crusted Salmon Fillets
- Snack: Energy-Boosting Nut and Seed Mix

DAY 2

- Breakfast: Nutrient-Packed Oatmeal Variation (use nuts and seeds instead of oats)
- Lunch: Wholesome Wrap and Sandwich Creation - Prosciutto-Wrapped Asparagus
- Dinner: Comforting Grain and Pasta Recipe - Zucchini Noodles with Pesto
- Snack: Guilt-Free Dip and Spread Recipe - Guacamole with Veggie Sticks

MEAL PLANNER

GLUTEN-FREE MEAL PLAN

DAY 1

- Breakfast: Energizing Smoothie Bowl (ensure all ingredients are gluten-free)
- Lunch: Colorful Grain Salad (use gluten-free grains)
- Dinner: Flavorful Fish and Seafood Dish - Herb-Crusted Salmon Fillets
- Snack: Energy-Boosting Nut and Seed Mix

DAY 2

- Breakfast: Nutrient-Packed Oatmeal Variation (use gluten-free oats)
- Lunch: Wholesome Wrap and Sandwich Creation - Stuffed Mushrooms with Cream Cheese and Spinach (ensure all ingredients are gluten-free)
- Dinner: Comforting Grain and Pasta Recipe - Garlic Parmesan Roasted Potatoes (use gluten-free breadcrumbs)
- Snack: Guilt-Free Dip and Spread Recipe - Hummus with Veggie Sticks

Paleo Meal Plan

DAY 1

- Breakfast: Protein-Packed Breakfast Burritos (use lettuce wraps instead of tortillas)
- Lunch: Satisfying Soup and Stew Recipe - Roasted Brussels Sprouts with Bacon
- Dinner: Flavorful Fish and Seafood Dish - Herb-Crusted Salmon Fillets
- Snack: Energy-Boosting Nut and Seed Mix

DAY 2

- Breakfast: Nutrient-Packed Oatmeal Variation (use nuts and seeds instead of oats)
- Lunch: Wholesome Wrap and Sandwich Creation - Prosciutto-Wrapped Asparagus
- Dinner: Comforting Grain and Pasta Recipe - Zucchini Noodles with Pesto
- Snack: Guilt-Free Dip and Spread Recipe - Guacamole with Veggie Sticks